KT-577-745

£25.3q

LANCHESTER LIBRARY

3 8001 00266 8204

A CLINICIAN'S GUIDE TO MENOPAUSE

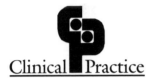

Clinical Practice

Judith H. Gold, M.D., F.R.C.P.C.
Elissa P. Benedek, M.D.
Series Editors

A CLINICIAN'S GUIDE TO MENOPAUSE

Edited by

Donna E. Stewart, M.D., F.R.C.P.C.
Gail Erlick Robinson, M.D., F.R.C.P.C.

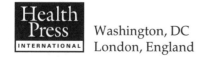

Washington, DC
London, England

Note: The authors have worked to ensure that all information in this book concerning drug dosages, schedules, and routes of administration is accurate as of the time of publication and consistent with standards set by the U.S. Food and Drug Administration and the general medical community. As medical research and practice advance, however, therapeutic standards may change. For this reason and because human and mechanical errors sometimes occur, we recommend that readers follow the advice of a physician who is directly involved in their care or the care of a member of their family.

Books published by the American Psychiatric Press, Inc., represent the views and opinions of the individual authors and do not necessarily represent the policies and opinions of the Press or the American Psychiatric Association.

Copyright © 1997 American Psychiatric Press, Inc.
ALL RIGHTS RESERVED
Manufactured in the United States of America on acid-free paper
First Edition   00   99   98   97   4   3   2   1

American Psychiatric Press, Inc.
1400 K Street, N.W., Washington, DC 20005
www.appi.org

Library of Congress Cataloging-in-Publication Data
A clinician's guide to menopause / edited by Donna E. Stewart and Gail
    Erlick Robinson. — 1st ed.
        p.   cm.
    Includes bibliographical references and index.
    ISBN 0-88048-754-2 (alk. paper)
    1. Menopause—Psychological aspects.   2. Menopause—Social
aspects.   3. Middle aged women—Psychology.   4. Middle aged
women—Mental health.   I. Stewart, Donna E., 1943–   .
II. Robinson, Gail Erlick, 1943–   .
    [DNLM: 1. Menopause—psychology.   2. Estrogen Replacement
Therapy—psychology.   3. Cross-Cultural Comparison.
WP 580 C641 1997]
RG186.C586   1997
612.6'65—dc21
DNLM/DLC
for Library of Congress   97-3185
                                                                   CIP

British Library Cataloguing in Publication Data
A CIP record is available from the British Library.

Coventry University

Contents

Contributors

David A. Baram, M.D.
Associate Professor of Obstetrics and Gynaecology and Psychiatry, The
University of Rochester School of Medicine and Dentistry, Rochester,
New York

Dara A. Charney, M.D., F.R.C.P.C.
Staff Psychiatrist, The Montreal General Hospital; and Assistant
Professor, Department of Psychiatry, McGill University, Montreal,
Quebec, Canada

Susan Feldman, M.A.
Director, Alma Unit on Women and Ageing, Key Centre for Women's
Health, The University of Melbourne, Carlton, Victoria, Australia

Leslie Hartley Gise, M.D.
Clinical Professor, Department of Psychiatry, John A. Burns School of
Medicine, University of Hawaii, Honolulu, Hawaii

Margaret F. Jensvold, M.D.
Director, Institute for Research on Women's Health; and private
psychiatric practice, Washington, D.C., and Bethesda, Maryland

John A. Lamont, M.Sc., M.D., F.R.C.S.C.
Professor, Obstetrics and Gynecology, McMaster University; and
Director, Sexual Medicine Unit, Henderson General Hospital,
Hamilton, Ontario, Canada

Harriette R. Mogul, M.D., M.P.H.
Chief, Section of Osteoporosis and Obesity, Division of Endocrinology
and Metabolism, New York Medical College; and Director, Menopausal
Health Program, Westchester County Medical Center, Valhalla, New
York

Yael Netz, Ph.D.
Visiting Fellow, Alma Unit on Women and Ageing, Key Centre for
Women's Health, The University of Melbourne, Carlton, Victoria,
Australia

Gail Erlick Robinson, M.D., F.R.C.P.C.
Director, Women's Mental Health Program, The Toronto Hospital;
Co-Director, Women's Mental Health Program, Department of
Psychiatry, University of Toronto; and Professor of Psychiatry,
Ob-Gyn, University of Toronto, Toronto, Ontario, Canada

Heather M. Shapiro, M.D., F.R.C.S.C.
Assistant Professor, Obstetrics/Gynecology, University of Toronto; and
Head, Mature Women's Clinic, The Toronto Hospital, Toronto,
Ontario, Canada

Donna E. Stewart, M.D., F.R.C.P.C.
Lillian Love Chair in Women's Health, Head of Women's Health, The
Toronto Hospital, Ontario Cancer Institute/Princess Margaret Hospital;
and Professor of Psychiatry, Ob-Gyn, Anesthesia, Surgery, Medicine,
Family and Community Medicine, University of Toronto, Toronto,
Ontario, Canada

Ruth Stirtzinger, M.D., F.R.C.P.C.
Staff Psychiatrist, Women's Clinic, The Toronto Hospital; and Assistant
Professor of Psychiatry, University of Toronto, Toronto, Ontario,
Canada

Nada L. Stotland, M.D.
Associate Professor, Departments of Psychiatry and
Obstetrics/Gynecology, The University of Chicago; and Diplomate,
Chicago Institute for Psychoanalysis, Chicago, Illinois

Gail G. Weber, B.Sc.N., M.Sc.
Coordinator of Programs for Midlife and Older Women/Menopause
Education, Regional Women's Health Centre, Women's College
Hospital, Toronto, Ontario, Canada

Introduction
to the Clinical Practice Series

Over the years of its existence the series of monographs entitled *Clinical Insights* gradually became focused on providing current, factual, and theoretical material of interest to the clinician working outside of a hospital setting. To reflect this orientation, the name of the Series has been changed to *Clinical Practice.*

The Clinical Practice Series will provide books that give the mental health clinician a practical, clinical approach to a variety of psychiatric problems. These books will provide up-to-date literature reviews and emphasize the most recent treatment methods. Thus, the publications in the Series will interest clinicians working both in psychiatry and in the other mental health professions.

Each year a number of books will be published dealing with all aspects of clinical practice. In addition, from time to time when appropriate, the publications may be revised and updated. Thus, the Series will provide quick access to relevant and important areas of psychiatric practice. Some books in the Series will be authored by a person considered to be an expert in that particular area; others will be edited by such an expert, who will also draw together other knowledgeable authors to produce a comprehensive overview of that topic.

Some of the books in the Clinical Practice Series will have their foundation in presentations at an annual meeting of the American Psychiatric Association. All will contain the most recently available information on the subjects discussed. Theoretical and scientific data will be applied to clinical situations, and case illustrations will be utilized in order to make the material even more relevant for the practitioner. Thus, the Clinical Practice Series should provide educational reading in a compact format especially designed for the mental health clinician–psychiatrist.

Judith H. Gold, M.D., F.R.C.P.C.
Series Editor

CHAPTER 1

Introduction

Donna E. Stewart, M.D., F.R.C.P.C.
Gail Erlick Robinson, M.D., F.R.C.P.C.

*T*he term *menopause* conjures up many contradictory associations: the loss of reproductive capacity *versus* freedom from pregnancy; the empty nest *versus* a child-free environment; a hormone depletion state *versus* a natural life transition; aging *versus* a new lease on life; symptoms *versus* wellness; and depression *versus* postmenopausal zest (Sherwin 1993).

Historically, women have been defined by their reproductive capacity, and, until the second half of the twentieth century, pregnancy often dominated their lives. However, with the advent of effective contraception, women achieved a much greater opportunity to develop identities defined by roles other than reproduction. Rapid social change has followed, and women now occupy positions in society undreamed of 50 years ago.

Women's health was also defined chiefly by reproduction. Women's health care was focused on problems related to "things down there" and was largely limited to matters of menstruation, fertility, pregnancy, and various gynecological misfortunes. Evidence-based practice was in even shorter supply than in the rest of medicine, and folklore and clinical anecdotal experience prevailed. Research on nonreproductive conditions and diseases was largely restricted to male subjects, and treatments derived from these studies were assumed to be equally applicable to women (Council on Ethical and Judicial Affairs, American Medical Association 1991).

What little research there was on women's health was chiefly concerned with pregnancy, and menopause was relatively neglected.

Menopause research initially had several problems, including the lack of a suitable definition of menopause itself. Some of this confusion has been abated by agreement on definition of terms. At the First International Congress on Menopause, menopause was described as the final menstrual period, which now occurs at an average age of 51 years. Menopause is retrospectively diagnosed 1 year after the permanent cessation of menses resulting from ovarian failure (Utian and Serr 1976). *Perimenopause,* or climacteric, is the phase in the female aging process marking the transition from the reproductive to the nonreproductive stages of life. It is sometimes, but not always, associated with symptoms and encompasses the time immediately before the cessation of menses and the first year afterward.

Menopause research was also confounded by the absence of criteria to determine whether menopause had occurred, because factors such as age, change in menstrual periods, presence of hot flashes, or direct measurement of hormones were sometimes used to make this diagnosis. Increasing rigor in studies has resulted in the use of standardized terms and more frequent measures of hormonal status. However, most of this research still occurs in women seeking medical treatment for symptoms attributed to menopause, and it is now known that these women differ from larger numbers of asymptomatic or mildly symptomatic women in the community.

The best available data were reported in a 5-year prospective, longitudinal, community-based study of 2,570 women's attitudes as they went through menopausal transition (McKinlay et al. 1992). The majority of women had positive feelings about menopause (42% felt relieved when menses stopped, and 35.5% reported neutral feelings). Whereas 19.6% of women reported mixed feelings about menopause, only 2.7% expressed regret. Negative feelings were more common in women who were depressed, had severe menopausal symptoms, or had previous negative expectations or attitudes about menopause.

Hormone studies of nonwhite women in other cultures, some of whom experience few, if any, symptoms at menopause, are still lacking.

Research into menopause has also been catalyzed by changes in population demographics and increasing interest in women's health. In addition, one must not forget market forces—there are enormous profits to be made on hormone replacement therapies, and this fuels research into pharmacological development. With advances in public health and better standards of living, the expected life span of both men and women has increased over the last century. Menopause is not new; there have always been women who, having survived the dangers of childhood and childbearing, lived long after menopause. What is new is the large proportion of women in the population who spend one-third to one-half of their lives after menopause. These numbers have been augmented by the aging baby boomers who are now reaching menopause. Women in general, and the baby boomers in particular, have become impatient with the lack of attention to women's health. As advocates of natural childbirth in the 1960s and 1970s are aging, they are now focusing on menopause.

Many feminists and other advocates argue that menopause is a natural life transition that has been medicalized and criticize the term *hormone replacement therapy,* which suggests a deficiency state. They also question the widespread recommendations for hormones and focus instead on the context of the woman's life and her empowerment. Increasing numbers of women advocate the use of natural remedies, which may include herbs, phytoestrogens, minerals, and other supplements, to assist in coping with menopausal symptoms. Unfortunately, although some of these unproven or traditional remedies may have value, no safety or efficacy studies have been done to date.

Other consumers and health care professionals note the positive effects of hormone replacement therapy in ameliorating short-term and long-term symptoms caused by the reduction in ovarian estrogen production and justify the term *replacement* as an accurate description of a treatment that aims to increase declining gonadal hormone levels. In this book, we use the term *hormone replacement therapy* for convenience and as a reflection of its aim to increase female sex hormone levels, and not as an endorsement of the medicalization of a natural life event in women.

Early research on menopause focused on comfort and the amelioration of transitional symptoms of lowered estrogen production by the ovary—hot flashes, night sweats, irregular menstrual periods, and urogenital atrophy. More recent research has focused on quality-of-life issues and the effects of estrogen on preventing cardiovascular disease and osteoporosis. When measured against possible long-term gains in disease prevention, symptom control during menopause has taken a back seat in the minds of researchers and physicians. However, many women are primarily motivated by a desire for symptom relief during menopausal transition and are reluctant to comply with long-term use in the face of varying estimates about prophylactic benefits for cardiovascular disease, perceived personal invulnerability to osteoporosis, and frightening data about increased risks for breast, ovarian, and endometrial cancer. Thus, clinicians and their patients may disagree about the optimal therapeutic course to follow during and after menopause. The fact that several popular magazines have featured articles on the pros and cons of hormone replacement therapy is a measure of a new interest in menopause and its controversies.

Psychiatry has also changed its perspective on menopause. Early diagnostic classifications from Kraepelin until DSM-III (American Psychiatric Association 1980) included involutional melancholia (a depressive disorder accompanied by agitation and delusions) as a separate disorder occurring in midlife. Although this condition was seen in both men and women, it was frequently attributed to menopause in women. Epidemiological data, however, fail to confirm an increase in severe depression or other mental disorders associated with menopause. Surveys conducted among women seeking medical care in menopause clinics, however, do show a high prevalence of anxiety and depression, and many of these women report previous depression often associated with reproductive events. Investigators increasingly hypothesize that a subgroup of women exists who are vulnerable to affective disorders at times of normal hormonal change (Stewart and Boydell 1993). Certainly, estrogen is known to have receptors in parts of the brain that regulate mood (see Chapters 6, 7, and 8). Serotonin deficiency is thought to be a causal factor in depression, and several mechanisms currently are described by which estrogen can enhance serotonergic neurotransmission. Many questions remain about depression; how to best treat it during menopause and the possible advantages of combining antidepressants with estrogen at menopause need further exploration (Pearce et al. 1995; Schmidt and Rubinow 1991).

Several books about menopause have been published recently. Some focus on the physiological and physical changes and the controversial role of hormone replacement; others emphasize the sociocultural or psychological perspective. In this book, we explore the rich multidimensional context of menopause from physiological, psychosocial, psychiatric, cross-cultural, sexual, and medical perspectives.

In Chapter 2, Baram reviews the physiology of menopause, including peri- and postmenopausal changes and the signs and symptoms of the climacteric.

In Chapter 3, Gise discusses the psychosocial aspects of menopause as a developmental life stage with issues related to the end of reproductivity, children, careers, marriages, and aging.

In Chapter 4, Weber explores the expression of menopausal symptoms in different cultures and discusses culturally sensitive approaches to menopausal health concerns.

In Chapter 5, Lamont addresses the issue of sexuality in the climacteric and postmenopausal years and reassures women that the normal physiological changes need not prevent a rich, satisfying sex life.

In Chapter 6, Mogul describes the medical evaluation of the perimenopausal woman, including the assessment of risk factors for cardiovascular disease, osteoporosis, and breast cancer, whereas in Chapter 7, Shapiro focuses on the treatment of various menopausal symptoms and examines the known risks and benefits of both hormonal and nonhormonal approaches.

In Chapter 8, Charney and Stewart describe the psychiatric aspects of menopause, noting the discrepancy between the assumption that menopause causes depression and the reality that most women do not have serious emotional disturbance at menopause.

In Chapter 9, Stotland provides an overview of psychological treatments available for women who do become emotionally distressed in the perimenopausal and menopausal stages of life, whereas in Chapter 10, Robinson and Stirtzinger focus specifically on the value of educational, psychodynamic, and self-help groups in ameliorating physical and emotional distress that may occur around the menopausal years.

In Chapter 11, Jensvold explores medication concerns for menopausal women, the effects of hormones on medications, and the effects of hormonal treatments on mood.

Finally, in Chapter 12, Feldman and Netz remind us that there is life after menopause and that the quality of life can be affected by expectations, relationships to society and the family, and attention to preventive health care.

We hope that by bringing these topics together in one book, a broader perspective of the menopausal transition will emerge to address a current gap in knowledge. We have written this book for clinicians (especially mental health practitioners) in the anticipation that they will find the physical and multidimensional context useful in their clinical work. Authors were selected from international authorities in psychiatry, gynecology, psychology, nursing, sociology, and internal medicine. Vignettes are included to illustrate common clinical problems and their resolution. We hope that this book will lead to future research on menopause, inform practitioners, and improve the care of women who seek help at this time of life.

References

American Psychiatric Association: Diagnostic and Statistical Manual of Mental Disorders, 3rd Edition. Washington, DC, American Psychiatric Association, 1980

Council on Ethical and Judicial Affairs, American Medical Association: Gender disparities in clinical decision making. JAMA 266:559–562, 1991

McKinlay SM, Brambilla DJ, Posner JG: The normal menopause transition. Maturitas 14:103–115, 1992

Pearce J, Hawtonk K, Blake F: Psychological and sexual symptoms associated with the menopause and the effects of hormone replacement therapy. Br J Psychiatry 167:163–173, 1995

Schmidt PJ, Rubinow DR: Menopause-related affective disorder: a justification for further study. Am J Psychiatry 148:844–852, 1991

Sherwin BB: Menopause: myths and realities in psychological aspects of women's health care, in The Interface Between Psychiatry and Obstetrics and Gynaecology. Edited by Stewart DE, Stotland NL. Washington, DC, American Psychiatric Press, 1993, pp 227–248

Stewart DE, Boydell KM: Psychological distress during menopause: associations across the reproductive life cycle. Int J Psychiatry Med 23:157–162, 1993

Utian WH, Serr D: The climacteric syndrome, in Consensus on Menopause Research. Edited by Van Keep PS, Greenblatt R, Fernet A. Lancaster, UK, MTP Press, 1976, pp 1–14

CHAPTER 2

Physiology and Symptoms of Menopause

David A. Baram, M.D.

As the older segment of the North American population continues to grow, health care providers will spend more of their time caring for elderly patients. North American women are living longer, and life expectancy, both at birth and at age 65, is increasing (Evans et al. 1993). Most women will live as many years after menopause (approximately 30 years, or about one-third of their life) as they did during their reproductive years. Because women outlive men by an average of 8 years (Evans et al. 1993), unmarried and unpartnered women now constitute a large portion of the elderly population. By age 85, women outnumber men by a ratio of more than 2 to 1 (Speroff 1994).

In this chapter, I review the following topics: 1) the age at which women begin to have symptoms of the perimenopause and menopause, 2) the endocrinology of the menopausal transition and how the diagnosis of menopause is made, 3) health maintenance for women during the climacteric, and 4) the physiological and anatomical changes caused by the postmenopausal decrease in estrogen production.

The author would like to thank Dr. Anthony Labrum for his help with preparation of the manuscript.

Age at Onset of Perimenopause and Menopause

The best data available on the age at onset of perimenopause and menopause come from the Massachusetts Women's Health Study (MWHS), a 5-year prospective, longitudinal, population-based study of 2,570 women (McKinlay et al. 1992). In addition to answers to questions about the age at onset of the perimenopause and menopause and the signs and symptoms of menopause, the MWHS recorded women's attitudes as they went through the menopausal transition. The MWHS found that the majority of women in the survey had positive feelings about menopause. Forty-two percent of the women in the study reported feeling relieved when menstruation ceased, and 35.5% reported neutral feelings. Some women (19.6%) reported mixed feelings about menopause, but only 2.7% of the women in the sample expressed regret when menstruation ceased. Negative feelings about menopause were more common in women who were depressed, had severe menopausal symptoms such as hot flashes and insomnia, or had previous negative attitudes and expectations about menopause.

Perimenopause is the phase in the climacteric aging process when women pass from reproductive to nonreproductive life (Jones and Muasher 1994). At this stage of life, the ovaries become relatively resistant to the stimulatory effects of the pituitary gonadotropins follicle-stimulating hormone (FSH) and luteinizing hormone (LH). During the perimenopause, women often have menstrual irregularity, longer and heavier menstrual periods, and prolonged episodes of amenorrhea. In addition to changes in the menstrual cycle, the perimenopause is marked by decreased (but not absent) fertility, vasomotor symptoms, psychological changes, insomnia, and changes in sexual function (Bachmann 1994a).

Data from the MWHS indicate that the perimenopausal transition usually begins about 4 years before complete cessation of menstrual periods (McKinlay et al. 1992; Speroff 1994) and that the median age at onset of perimenopause is 47.5 years. In the MWHS, smokers were noted to have a shorter perimenopause than nonsmokers (McKinlay et al. 1992). Most women in the MWHS (90%) noted menstrual irregularity for years before their last menstrual period; the other 10% had less than 6 months of menstrual irregularity before menopause or noted that their periods stopped abruptly and without warning (McKinlay et al. 1992).

Menopause is the time in a woman's life when, after the depletion or atrophy of all gonadotropin-sensitive ovarian follicles, menstruation permanently ceases. Menopause—defined as 12 consecutive months of amenorrhea usually accompanied by hot flashes and urogenital atrophy—is usually diagnosed retrospectively on a clinical basis, after the woman has experienced her final menstrual period. Elevated FSH concentrations (>40 IU/L) are commonly used to confirm the diagnosis of menopause, but recent studies (Burger 1994) have reported that postmenopausal concentrations of FSH can be found in regularly cycling perimenopausal women. Therefore, menopause cannot be diagnosed solely on the basis of an elevated concentration of FSH (Barnes and Hajj 1993).

In the MWHS, the median age at onset of menopause was 51.3 years (range, 47–55 years). Although the median age at onset of menarche has decreased significantly worldwide as a result of improved nutrition and better health care, the age at onset of menopause has remained the same since the time of ancient Greece (Speroff 1994). The MWHS found that women who currently smoke experience menopause 1.5 years earlier than women who do not smoke. There is evidence of a dose-response relationship between the age at onset of menopause and the number of cigarettes smoked and duration of smoking. Former smokers and women who live at high altitudes also have an earlier onset of menopause (Midgette and Baron 1990; Speroff 1994). Cigarette smoking may cause an earlier onset of menopause by 1) exerting a direct toxic effect on ovarian follicles, 2) interfering with the hypothalamic-pituitary-ovarian axis, or 3) affecting the metabolism of the reproductive hormones (Midgette and Baron 1990). Oral contraceptives, marital status, race, geographic location (except for women living at high altitudes), parity, age at onset of menarche, mother's age at onset of menopause, height, hormone replacement therapy, and socioeconomic status (level of education and income) do not affect the age at onset of menopause (Avis and McKinlay 1995). Thin or malnourished women have an earlier onset of menopause, probably because they have less body fat available for the peripheral conversion of androstenedione to estrogen.

Menopause occurs before age 40 in about 1% of women. This condition is known as *premature ovarian failure* and is usually idiopathic. However, in rare cases, premature ovarian failure can be caused by autoimmune disease (especially thyroid disease) or is associated with myasthenia gravis, idiopathic thrombocytopenic purpura, rheumatoid arthritis, vitiligo, or autoimmune hemolytic anemia (Speroff et al. 1994). Occasionally, younger women may experience oligomenorrhea, menopausal symptoms, and infertility because of a diminished number of ovarian follicles. In these patients, FSH concentrations may be in the menopausal range (>40 IU/L) temporarily. Some of these women may begin to menstruate and ovulate again, however, and may eventually become pregnant. When these patients resume menstruation, their FSH concentrations return to the premenopausal range.

Endocrinology of Menopause

Perimenopausal Changes

Changes in the concentration and ratio of the reproductive hormones begin many years before menopause and are probably caused by several factors. The primary factor is a decrease in the number of functioning ovarian follicles as a result of ovarian atresia. The number of ovarian follicles decreases from an estimated high of 7 million during embryonic life to about 2 million at birth. Of the remaining follicles, about 400 to 500 are ovulated during the reproductive period of life, and the remainder are lost through atresia. Other factors that lead to changes in reproductive hormones during perimenopause include resistance of the remaining ovarian follicles to gonadotropin stimulation (the "better" or more responsive ovarian follicles may be used earlier in life) and alterations in the sensitivity of the hypothalamic-pituitary-ovarian axis to changing estrogen concentrations (Longcope 1994; Metcalf et al. 1982; Speroff et al. 1994). Perimenopausal hormonal changes often begin during the mid-30s and are partially responsible for the decreased fertility noted by women in their 30s and 40s (Schinfeld 1994). In addition, as women age, their menstrual cycles increase in length, become more irregular (menstrual cycles are most regular during middle reproductive life), and are often anovulatory (Hee et al. 1993; Speroff et al. 1994).

The first detectable hormonal change of the perimenopause is a rising concentration of FSH and a declining concentration of inhibin (Jones and Muasher 1994; Sherman et al. 1976). The rising FSH concentration is probably caused by a decrease in the number of gonadotropin-sensitive ovarian follicles, which stimulates the pituitary gland to produce more FSH in an effort to stimulate the resistant follicles. At the same time, the circulating concentrations of inhibin and, to a lesser extent, estradiol decrease. Inhibin, a sensitive measure of ovarian function, is produced by the granulosa cells surrounding the ovarian follicles. Inhibin and estrogen both have a negative feedback effect on FSH, and as the aging ovary produces less inhibin and estradiol, the amount of FSH produced by the pituitary gland increases. The production of inhibin begins to decrease at about age 35 and stops completely at menopause (Hee et al. 1993).

During the early perimenopausal phase, while FSH is increasing and inhibin is decreasing, the concentration of LH remains in the normal range. Late in the perimenopause, LH concentrations increase slightly but at a slower rate than that of FSH. The concentration of estrogen (primarily estradiol) remains in the normal range until approximately 3 years before menopause, when it gradually begins to decline (MacNaughton et al. 1992; Trevoux et al. 1986). Once menopause has occurred and all of the ovarian follicles have been depleted, estrogen concentrations decline precipitously.

Later in the perimenopause, FSH concentrations continue to rise, which has a significant effect on the menstrual cycle. The elevated FSH concentrations noted during the early follicular stage of each perimenopausal menstrual cycle cause unusually rapid follicular development and a relative decrease in the concentration of circulating follicular-phase estrogen. In addition, the follicular phase of the menstrual cycle becomes shorter. In the late perimenopausal phase, as transitory ovarian failure occurs, menstrual cycles become increasingly irregular, and many of the cycles become anovulatory. At this time, luteal phase defects caused by decreased progesterone production by the corpus luteum are common, and conception becomes increasingly rare.

As noted earlier in this chapter, elevated—or postmenopausal—concentrations of FSH and LH and decreased concentrations of estradiol and progesterone can be detected before ovarian function ceases permanently (Hee et al. 1993). In other words, the hormonal profile of perimenopausal women during times of prolonged amenorrhea can be similar to the hormonal profile of postmenopausal women (Burger 1994; Hee et al. 1993). Therefore, perimenopausal women with elevated FSH concentrations can still become pregnant, and they should be cautioned to use birth control to avoid unplanned pregnancy until both LH and FSH concentrations are consistently and permanently elevated.

Postmenopausal Changes

With the onset of menopause, ovarian production of estrogen (both estradiol and estrone), progesterone, androstenedione, and testosterone decreases significantly. Estrogen concentrations decline significantly once menstruation ceases permanently, which leads to atrophy of estrogen-sensitive tissue (i.e., breast, bladder, skin, and internal and external genitalia). The loss of the negative feedback of estrogen on the pituitary gland leads to a dramatic increase in the production of FSH and LH as the gonadotropins attempt to stimulate the unresponsive ovarian follicles. In postmenopausal women, FSH production increases 10- to 20-fold and LH production increases 3-fold. Gonadotropin concentrations reach maximum levels 1–3 years after menopause and then decrease slowly during the remaining postmenopausal years (Speroff et al. 1994).

After all of the ovarian follicles have been depleted, the ovary stops producing significant amounts of estrogen. However, the stroma of the postmenopausal ovary is stimulated by high levels of gonadotropins and continues to produce testosterone and smaller amounts of androstenedione (Longcope 1994). Most estrogen found in postmenopausal women is derived from the peripheral conversion of adrenal (70%) and ovarian (30%) androstenedione to estrone. Estradiol is the primary estrogen found in women during the reproductive years, whereas estrone is the primary estrogen noted in postmenopausal women. Some of the estrone produced by the peripheral conversion of androstenedione is converted to estradiol. The peripheral conversion of androstenedione to estrogens by aromatization takes place primarily in adipose tissue but also occurs in muscle, skin, and the liver. Therefore, overweight or obese women are hyperestrogenic when compared with thin women and are more likely to develop estrogen-dependent neoplasia, especially adenocarcinoma of the endometrium (Speroff et al. 1994). After menopause, there is no further corpus luteum formation, and the ovary no longer produces progesterone. The small amount of progesterone detectable in postmenopausal women is secreted exclusively by the adrenal gland (Metcalf et al. 1982).

In addition to the testosterone produced by the ovary, androgens are produced by the postmenopausal adrenal gland. The amount of androgen (androstenedione and testosterone) produced by the adrenal gland decreases after menopause. After menopause, estrogen production declines more significantly than androgen production, and, for this reason, the androgen-to-estrogen ratio changes significantly in postmenopausal women. This change in the androgen-to-estrogen ratio may be responsible for the facial hirsutism and loss of scalp hair noted by some postmenopausal women (Gass 1993; Speroff et al. 1994).

Toward the end of life, androstenedione production by the adrenal gland decreases significantly. In turn, little estrogen is produced by peripheral conversion of androgens, and estrogen-responsive tissue atrophies further.

Health Maintenance

The annual well-patient visit is an excellent opportunity for health care providers to screen perimenopausal and menopausal women for medical disorders and to counsel them about preventive health care. The physician should take a complete history, do a physical examination, and order appropriate laboratory studies during the annual visit (American College of Obstetrics and Gynaecology 1995).

The patient history should include questions about menopausal symptoms, medication use (both prescription and over the counter), diet, physical activity level, substance use and abuse, smoking, domestic violence, injury prevention, sexuality, mental health (especially symptoms of depression), and psychosocial factors (e.g., relationships, work, home environment, and children). The physician should discuss pregnancy concerns and contraception with perimenopausal women (American College of Obstetrics and Gynaecology 1995). The physician should also obtain a complete family history, with special attention to a family history of cardiovascular disease, osteoporosis, diabetes, cancer, hypertension, and depression, as well as review the patient's immunization history and update immunizations as needed.

The physical examination of perimenopausal or postmenopausal women should include measurements of height (postmenopausal women lose height due to osteoporosis), weight, and blood pressure; tests of visual and auditory acuity; and a thorough examination of the oral cavity, skin, neck, breasts, abdomen, pelvis, and rectum, including a stool sample to test for occult blood. The clinician should use care when inserting a speculum during the pelvic examination, especially in postmenopausal women. The smallest well-lubricated speculum should be inserted, especially in women who are not sexually active. A gentle bimanual vaginal and rectovaginal examination should be done, placing only one finger in the vagina.

Laboratory tests should routinely include an annual Papanicolaou (Pap) smear, mammography (every 2 years after age 40 and annually beginning at age 50), cholesterol screening (every 5 years), and sigmoidoscopy (every 5 years beginning at age 50). The timing and frequency of these screening tests may vary depending on family history and the appearance of symptoms. Thyroid disease and diabetes are more common in perimenopausal and menopausal women than in premenopausal women, and screening for these conditions should be considered when there is a family history of these disorders or when the patient is symptomatic.

Symptoms of Menopausal Transition

Symptoms frequently noted by women undergoing the menopausal transition include

- Urogenital atrophy causing dyspareunia, vulvar itching, and urinary difficulties (e.g., urethritis, urge incontinence, and urinary frequency)
- Vasomotor instability (or hot flashes), often contributing to insomnia
- Irregular menstrual bleeding

Many women report that irregular menstrual bleeding and episodes of amenorrhea are the most distressing symptoms of perimenopause (McKinlay et al. 1992). In addition, perimenopausal and menopausal women often report a number of general physical and emotional symptoms. These symptoms occur more frequently in women who experience hot flashes, especially if they are severe. Physical symptoms include headaches, breast sensitivity, weight gain, thinning of the skin, dizziness, palpitations, and muscle and joint pain. Emotional symptoms include (in order of decreasing frequency) irritability, fatigue, tension, nervousness, depression, lack of motivation, insomnia (or early-morning awakening), and feelings of isolation (Anderson et al. 1987; Oldenhave and Netelenbos 1994; Oldenhave et al. 1993). It is difficult to determine whether these symptoms are caused by hormonal or psychosocial factors.

Vulvovaginal Symptoms and Anatomical Changes

Common vulvovaginal symptoms found in postmenopausal women include irritation, itching, burning, and dyspareunia caused by vaginal atrophy. A chronic vaginal discharge caused by a change in the vaginal environment from acidic to alkaline is common during menopause. Extensive vulvovaginal atrophy often causes bleeding, sometimes with only a light touch. A sensation of pressure in the vagina and pelvis may be caused by a cystocele, a rectocele, an enterocele, or uterine prolapse. Aging results in loss of skin collagen and subcutaneous fat, which causes wrinkling of the skin and thinning of the labia majora and mons pubis. Loss and thinning of pubic hair are also common. Although most of the vulvovaginal symptoms noted above are due to urogenital atrophy, more serious conditions always must be ruled out. The differential diagnosis of pelvic bleeding, pain, pressure, or burning should in-

clude benign and malignant neoplasms, vulvar dystrophies, infections, trauma, foreign bodies, and allergic reactions (Bachmann
1994b).

Both the vulva and the vagina contain a rich supply of estrogen
receptors (Waggoner 1993). Therefore, vulvovaginal atrophy begins during the perimenopausal years as estrogen levels begin to
wane. The vulva of peri- and postmenopausal women loses collagen and adipose tissue and becomes thinner, flattened, and less
elastic (Bachmann 1994a). The secretions of the vulvar sebaceous
glands diminish, and the clitoris becomes smaller and less sensitive
to touch. The prepuce of the clitoris atrophies, which causes clitoral
irritation when the clitoris is stimulated during sexual arousal and
intercourse. Many women notice that the dryness, irritation, burning, and itching caused by vulvar atrophy make them uncomfortable during the day and interfere with sleep at night.

The postmenopausal vagina loses rugae and becomes smooth
and atrophic, and the vaginal walls appear smooth, friable, and
pale. The alkaline vaginal environment and loss of glycogen from
the vagina do not support the growth of the lactobacilli commonly
found in the acidic premenopausal vagina; thus, postmenopausal
women are more susceptible to vaginal infections (Bachmann
1994b; Gass 1993). Because the vascularity and the collagen content
of the vagina decrease and the mucosa thins, the vagina becomes
more friable and more susceptible to trauma and infection. The
vagina loses length, diameter, and distensibility. These structural
changes, along with the decrease in the amount of vaginal lubrication produced during sexual arousal, make dyspareunia a common
problem in the elderly. Regular use of vaginal estrogen cream may
reduce burning, itching, and dyspareunia. Use of lubricants before
intercourse may also be helpful for dyspareunia.

Because of the friability of the vaginal mucosa, bleeding is common whenever the vaginal mucosa is traumatized, such as during
speculum insertion or intercourse. Again, the clinician must thoroughly investigate any vulvovaginal bleeding to rule out vaginal,
vulvar, cervical, and endometrial neoplasms. As the postmenopausal vagina undergoes anatomical changes, the urethral meatus
moves closer to the introitus, often resulting in dysuria, urinary
frequency and urgency, and urinary tract infections.

As estrogen levels decline with the cessation of menses, the endometrium becomes atrophic, and the uterus and cervix decrease significantly in size. These anatomical changes occur gradually over time and continue throughout the lifetime of the woman. Uterine fibroids, which are dependent on estrogen stimulation for growth, often diminish dramatically postmenopause. Therefore, women with symptomatic uterine fibroids may want to delay surgical treatment until the effect of menopause on the size of the fibroids can be assessed. The cervical os becomes stenotic, and the transformation zone of the cervix moves upward into the endocervical canal, making it more difficult to obtain sufficient cellular material for a Pap smear. Provided the cervix is not too stenotic, an adequate Pap smear can be obtained if a small endocervical brush is placed high in the endocervical canal.

After menopause, the ovaries decrease significantly in size and are barely palpable during bimanual examination. Because postmenopausal women are anovulatory, functional cysts (corpus luteum cysts and follicular cysts) should not form in the ovaries. Therefore, any mass in the ovaries of postmenopausal women must be further evaluated to rule out the possibility of ovarian carcinoma.

The breasts of postmenopausal women lose support and subcutaneous fat, decrease in size, and lie flatter against the chest wall (Gass 1993). Breast parenchyma is eventually totally replaced with fatty tissue. The breast areola also decreases in size after menopause.

The estrogen deprivation that occurs at the onset of menopause can contribute to a decrease in the strength of the connective tissue and muscles supporting the uterus, bladder, and rectum (Hajj 1993). As women age, the ligaments supporting the pelvic viscera become more lax, allowing uterine prolapse (procidentia), cystocele, enterocele, and rectocele to develop. These anatomical changes, which are more common in multiparous women, may eventually cause pelvic pressure and discomfort, stress urinary incontinence, and difficulty emptying the bowel. Stress urinary incontinence can cause significant changes in a woman's lifestyle, leading to social withdrawal and isolation, avoidance of lovemaking, and curtailment of physical activity. When bathroom facilities are not readily available, women with urinary incontinence may have difficulty traveling, working, and shopping. Women with incontinence often must carefully plan trips away from home and must carry a change of clothing and locate bathrooms ahead of time. Common emotional responses to incontinence include depression, guilt, denial, anxiety, secretiveness, and fear that others will discover the patient's difficulty or smell the urine (Thiede 1992).

Hot Flashes

Hot flashes (or flushes) are the most reliable indicator of menopause, the most frequently reported menopausal symptom (Swartzman et al. 1990), and one of the most distressing symptoms for perimenopausal and menopausal women (Kronenberg 1994). A hot flash is "a sudden, transient sensation ranging from warmth to intense heat that spreads over the body, particularly on the chest, face, and head, typically accompanied by flushing, perspiration, and often followed by a chill. In some instances, there are palpitations, and feelings of anxiety" (Kronenberg 1994, p. 97). In addition, some women experience vertigo and weakness during a hot flash (Ginsburg 1994). Many women experience an aura or prodromal sensation consisting of anxiety, tingling, or head pressure that precedes the hot flash by 5–60 seconds.

Significant risk factors for menopausal hot flashes include earlier age at onset of menopause, surgical menopause, and less than 12 years of education (McKinlay et al. 1992; Schwingl et al. 1994). Past or current alcohol consumption places women at higher risk for developing hot flashes. In the MWHS (McKinlay et al. 1992), no statistically significant association between cigarette smoking and hot flashes was found. Heavier women were less likely than thin women to experience hot flashes, probably because of enhanced perimenopausal and postmenopausal estrogen production. Thin women who smoked during the perimenopause were most likely to experience hot flashes during menopause. Race, parity, and age at first and last pregnancy were not related to hot flashes at the time of menopause (Schwingl et al. 1994). In the MWHS (McKinlay et al. 1992), women who had fewer general physical symptoms before menopause and more positive attitudes toward menopause were less likely to report hot flashes.

What causes hot flashes? Although no exact etiology has been found, one hypothesis (Kronenberg 1994) suggested that changes in the thermoregulatory system located in the hypothalamus are most likely responsible. At the beginning of a hot flash, the body's thermostat undergoes a temporary downward resetting, making the body feel warmer than it actually is. The woman responds by attempting to cool down through sweating, cutaneous vasodilatation, and changes in behavior leading to a cooler environment. Once core body cooling takes place, the setting of the hypothalamic thermostat returns to normal and the woman conserves heat until core body temperature is again normal. The substance responsible for resetting the body's thermostat during a hot flash is unknown, but possibilities include the sex steroids and the opioid peptides (Kronenberg 1994).

The role of estrogen and other hormones and centrally acting neurotransmitters in the etiology of hot flashes is unknown. However, the association of estrogen deficiency with hot flashes can be inferred from the impressive effectiveness of estrogen replacement therapy (ERT) for hot flashes. Although most hot flashes are temporally associated with an increase in gonadotropin-releasing hormone (GnRH) and LH levels, there does not seem to be a causal relationship between the pulsatile release of GnRH and/or LH and the onset of a hot flash. Indeed, hot flashes can occur in women who have had hypophysectomies. Other hormonal changes that have been noted when hot flashes occur include increases in plasma levels of epinephrine, β-endorphin, adrenocorticotropic hormone (ACTH), cortisol, dehydroepiandrosterone, and androstenedione. However, none of these hormonal changes has been shown to precipitate hot flashes (Kronenberg 1994).

The sweating noted at the start of a hot flash usually is accompanied by an increase in finger temperature, a decrease in skin resistance, and an increase in skin conductance (Kronenberg 1994; Swartzman et al. 1990). At times, sweating can be profuse, causing clothing to become literally soaked. Heart rate, cutaneous blood flow, and skin temperature increase during the hot flash, but blood pressure does not change significantly. Cutaneous vasodilatation (which is responsible for the "flush"), sweating, and attempts by the woman to cool off (e.g., taking off clothing, opening windows, moving to a cooler environment) cause heat loss and a slight lowering of core body temperature, often precipitating a chilling sensation, vasoconstriction, and actual shivering. Skin temperature then gradually returns to normal, often taking as long as 30 minutes (Kronenberg 1994).

A hot flash lasts from several seconds to a few minutes (Speroff et al. 1994). The frequency of hot flashes and the way in which hot flashes are experienced also vary, both within and among individual women (Kronenberg 1994). Some women sweat profusely, whereas others do not. Symptoms in any woman may, of course, change over time. Hot flashes often occur spontaneously without any obvious precipitant; however, they can be triggered in some women by psychological stress, hot and humid weather, caffeine, alcohol, or certain foods (Kronenberg 1994).

Most American women experience hot flashes during the menopausal transition (Avis and McKinlay 1995; McKinlay et al. 1992; Schwingl et al. 1994). However, in the MWHS, 23% of the postmenopausal women never had hot flashes or night sweats. The prevalence of hot flashes can vary considerably depending on the population studied. Japanese women, who have been studied extensively, rarely report hot flashes, perhaps because of cultural expectations or the plant estrogen they receive naturally from their diet (Lock et al. 1988).

Women often report hot flashes before the onset of menopause. The MWHS (Avis and McKinlay 1995; McKinlay et al. 1992) found that 10% of women had hot flashes before the onset of menstrual irregularity. The peak time for reporting hot flashes, when they were experienced by 50% of the women in the study, occurred late in the perimenopause, just prior to the onset of menopause. Women in the MWHS who did have hot flashes noted that they were most prevalent during the first 2 years after menopause and that they decreased over time. Only 20% of the women in the MWHS were still experiencing hot flashes 4 years after their final menstrual period. Women with a perimenopause of less than 6 months (about 10% of the MWHS sample) had a much lower prevalence of hot flashes—about 30%—than did women with a longer perimenopause.

The majority of women in the MWHS who experienced hot flashes (69%) reported that they were not bothered by them. Only 32% of the women in the study consulted a physician for treatment of menopausal symptoms, usually because their hot flashes or night sweats were frequent, were severe, and caused insomnia. However, hot flashes, especially those that are severe and persist for a long time, can be quite troublesome and embarrassing for some women. Women often need to modify their behavior or environment (e.g., wearing light clothing or changing the room temperature) to accommodate the profuse sweating that accompanies hot flashes.

Women who have hot flashes are often awakened at night and are twice as likely to report insomnia as women who do not have hot flashes (Erlik et al. 1981). Women who have difficulty sleeping because of hot flashes often report irritability and fatigue the next day (Shaver et al. 1988). Insomnia caused by hot flashes is the primary reason that women seek medical care and ERT during the menopausal transition (Kronenberg 1994). The beneficial effects of ERT on sleep include reduction in insomnia, shorter time to get to sleep (sleep latency), and fewer episodes of wakefulness during the night. In addition, ERT in women with hot flashes increases the amount of time spent in deeper and more restful rapid eye movement (REM) sleep (Erlik et al. 1981; Schiff et al. 1979). With improved sleep patterns, women report less anxiety and improved ability to function socially (Schiff et al. 1979). (Other treatment approaches to hot flashes are reviewed by Shapiro, Chapter 7, in this volume.)

Irregular Menstrual Bleeding

During the perimenopausal transition, changes in the typical menstrual cycle pattern often occur. Some women may develop dysfunctional or anovulatory uterine bleeding, which is characterized by irregular menstrual periods (metrorrhagia), intermenstrual spotting, excessive and prolonged menstrual periods (menorrhagia), and episodes of amenorrhea. Dysfunctional uterine bleeding implies that the bleeding comes from the endometrium and is not caused by a neoplastic process in the endometrial cavity or by a medical illness (Speroff et al. 1994). Shortened menstrual cycle intervals may be caused by a decrease in the length of the follicular phase of the cycle (Gass 1993). Most of the perimenopausal changes in the menstrual cycle are due to anovulation. If ovulation does not occur, no corpus luteum is formed, and no progesterone is available to bring about secretory changes to the endometrium. High sustained levels of estrogen, unopposed by the effects of progesterone, can cause an abnormal thickening of endometrial tissue that eventually leads to irregular ripening and shedding of the endometrium. After many years, unopposed estrogen stimulation of the endometrium can result in adenomatous hyperplasia or endometrial carcinoma (Speroff et al. 1994).

Slight changes in the duration or amount of menstrual blood flow may be normal, but any significant changes in the menstrual pattern require evaluation to rule out a benign or malignant neoplastic process of the upper or lower genital tract. Abnormal bleeding also can be related to pregnancy or a medical illness, such as a clotting abnormality. Although fertility decreases significantly during the perimenopause, health care providers should always consider the possibility of pregnancy in premenopausal women with abnormal bleeding. Any postmenopausal bleeding must be considered an endometrial carcinoma until proven otherwise and should be evaluated as soon as possible with an endometrial curettage. The most convenient and least painful way to evaluate dysfunctional uterine bleeding or postmenopausal bleeding is to perform an office endometrial aspiration curettage. This simple procedure usually can be done with local anesthesia and is as accurate as an in-hospital dilatation and curettage (Speroff et al. 1994). Other modalities for evaluating the endometrium include hysteroscopy (especially valuable for visualizing endometrial polyps) and visualization of the endometrium with vaginal ultrasound.

After any neoplastic process has been ruled out, perimenopausal anovulatory uterine bleeding can be managed with the administration of a short course of progesterone alone (either in oral or in intramuscular depo form) or continuous daily administration of an estrogen/progesterone combination. In low-risk perimenopausal women (i.e., those who do not smoke, do not have a dyslipidemia, and are not hypertensive), a low-dose oral contraceptive can also be used and is a good choice if contraception is desired. Women who continue to bleed with the above regimen should consider a trial of danocrine or the intramuscular depo form of a GnRH agonist. If medical therapy fails to control dysfunctional uterine bleeding, endomyometrial ablation or hysterectomy is a possible last resort.

Conclusion

The median age at onset of menopause is 51.3 years, with perimenopause beginning about 4 years earlier. Decreases in the number of functioning ovarian follicles, increased resistance of the remaining follicles to gonadotropin stimulation, and alterations in the sensitivity of the hypothalamic-pituitary-ovarian axis to changing estrogen concentrations all contribute to the changes in the concentrations and ratios of the reproductive hormones that herald the beginning of menopause. Symptoms reported include dyspareunia and urinary difficulties due to urogenital atrophy, vasomotor instability (hot flashes), and irregular menstrual bleeding. Management of these symptoms is further discussed in Chapters 5 and 7.

References

American College of Obstetrics and Gynaecology: Health maintenance for perimenopausal women. ACOG Technical Bulletin 210:1–10, August 1995

Anderson E, Hamburger S, Liu JH, et al: Characteristics of menopausal women seeking assistance. Am J Obstet Gynecol 156:428–433, 1987

Avis NE, McKinlay SM: The Massachusetts Women's Health Study: an epidemiologic investigation of the menopause. J Am Med Wom Assoc 50:45–63, 1995

Bachmann GA: The changes before "the change." Postgrad Med 95:113–124, 1994a

Bachmann GA: Vulvovaginal complaints, in Treatment of the Postmenopausal Woman: Basic and Clinical Aspects. Edited by Lobo RA. New York, Raven, 1994b, pp 137–142

Barnes R, Hajj SN: Pathophysiology of menopause, in Clinical Reproductive Gynaecology. Edited by Hajj SN, Evans WJ. Norwalk, CT, Appleton & Lange, 1993, pp 31–35

Burger HG: The menopause: when it is all over or is it? Aust N Z J Obstet Gynaecol 34:293–295, 1994

Erlik Y, Tataryn IV, Meldrum DR, et al: Association of waking episodes with menopausal hot flushes. JAMA 245:1741–1744, 1981

Evans WJ, Evans MI, Hajj SN: The aging population, in Clinical Reproductive Gynaecology. Edited by Hajj SN, Evans WJ. Norwalk, CT, Appleton & Lange, 1993, pp 1–12

Gass M: Physiology and pathophysiology of the postmenopausal years, in Gynaecology and Obstetrics: A Longitudinal Approach. Edited by Moore TR, Reiter RC, Rebar RW, et al. New York, Churchill Livingstone, 1993, pp 883–896

Ginsburg ES: Hot flashes—physiology, hormonal therapy, and alternative therapies. Obstet Gynecol Clin North Am 21:381–390, 1994

Hajj SN: Pelvic relaxation and procidentia, in Clinical Reproductive Gynaecology. Edited by Hajj SN, Evans WJ. Norwalk, CT, Appleton & Lange, 1993, pp 112–117

Hee J, MacNaughton J, Bangah M, et al: Perimenopausal patterns of gonadotrophins, immunoreactive inhibin, oestradiol and progesterone. Maturitas 18:9–20, 1993

Jones GS, Muasher SJ: Hormonal changes in the perimenopause, in The Menopause: Comprehensive Management, 3rd Edition. Edited by Eskin BA. New York, McGraw-Hill, 1994, pp 257–268

Kronenberg F: Hot flashes, in Treatment of the Postmenopausal Woman: Basic and Clinical Aspects. Edited by Lobo RA. New York, Raven, 1994, pp 97–117

Lock M, Kaufert P, Gilbert P: Cultural construction of the menopausal syndrome: the Japanese case. Maturitas 10:317–332, 1988

Longcope C: The endocrinology of the menopause, in Treatment of the Postmenopausal Woman: Basic and Clinical Aspects. Edited by Lobo RA. New York, Raven, 1994, pp 47–53

MacNaughton J, Banah M, McCloud P, et al: Age related changes in follicle stimulating hormone, luteinizing hormone, oestradiol and immunoreactive inhibin in women of reproductive age. Clin Endocrinol (Oxf) 36:339–345, 1992

McKinlay SM, Brambilla DJ, Posner JG: The normal menopause transition. Maturitas 14:103–115, 1992

Metcalf MG, Donald RA, Livesey JH: Pituitary-ovarian function before, during and after the menopause: a longitudinal study. Clin Endocrinol (Oxf) 17:489–494, 1982

Midgette AS, Baron JA: Cigarette smoking and the risk of natural menopause. Epidemiology 1:475–480, 1990

Oldenhave A, Netelenbos C: Pathogenesis of climacteric complaints: ready for the change? Lancet 343:649–653, 1994

Oldenhave A, Jaszmann JB, Haspels AA, et al: Impact of climacteric on well-being. Am J Obstet Gynecol 168:772–780, 1993

Schiff I, Regestein Q, Tulchinsky D, et al: Effects of estrogens on sleep and psychological state of hypogonadal women. JAMA 242:2405–2407, 1979

Schinfeld JS: Sex steroid hormone metabolism in the climacteric woman, in The Menopause: Comprehensive Management, 3rd Edition. Edited by Eskin BA. New York, McGraw-Hill, 1994, pp 269–288

Schwingl PJ, Hulka BS, Harlow SD: Risk factors for menopausal hot flashes. Obstet Gynecol 84:29–34, 1994

Shaver J, Giblin E, Lentz M, et al: Sleep patterns and stability in perimenopausal women. Sleep 11:556–561, 1988

Sherman BM, West JH, Korenman SG: The menopausal transition: analysis of LH, FSH, estradiol, and progesterone concentrations during menstrual cycles of older women. J Clin Endocrinol Metab 42:629–636, 1976

Speroff L: The menopause: a signal for the future, in Treatment of the Postmenopausal Woman: Basic and Clinical Aspects. Edited by Lobo RA. New York, Raven, 1994, pp 1–8

Speroff L, Glass RH, Kase NG: Clinical Gynecologic Endocrinology and Infertility, 5th Edition. Baltimore, MD, Williams & Wilkins, 1994

Swartzman LC, Edelberg R, Kemmann E: The menopausal hot flush: symptom reports and concomitant physiological changes. J Behav Med 13:15–30, 1990

Thiede HA: Psychosocial factors, in Female Pelvic Floor Disorders: Investigation and Management. Edited by Benson JT. New York, WW Norton, 1992, pp 179–184

Trevoux R, DeBrux J, Castanier M, et al: Endometrium and plasma hormone profile in the peri-menopause and post-menopause. Maturitas 8:309–326, 1986

Waggoner SE: Vulva and vagina, in Clinical Reproductive Gynaecology. Edited by Hajj SN, Evans WJ. Norwalk, CT, Appleton & Lange, 1993, pp 159–176

CHAPTER 3

Psychosocial Aspects

Leslie Hartley Gise, M.D.

Although the tendency is to attribute all midlife symptoms to menopause, the fact that some women have no symptoms highlights the distinction between what is inevitable or biological and what is environmental, which includes psychological, social, and cultural factors. Confusion of causation with association has interfered with the understanding of the psychosocial aspects of menopause (Schmidt and Rubinow 1991). Symptoms and psychosocial concerns related to aging and midlife have been mistakenly attributed to the end of reproductive capacity.

Sociocultural Factors

Loss of Status

In Western society, a woman's identity has been derived from the status and characteristics of the men in her life (Notman 1995). Until the 1980 census, a woman's socioeconomic status was determined by that of her husband or of her father. Because a woman's identity has been viewed largely in relation to her reproductive status as the mother of children, the potential mother of children, or a woman who is no longer able to have children, the loss of fertility at menopause may affect a woman's social position achieved during her reproductive years (Notman 1995). For women who never had children, midlife finalizes this reality and may activate past conflicts that had seemed resolved. Women who did not actively make the decision not to have children may have difficulty facing the reality of their childlessness at midlife.

Aging

Although menopause occurs at midlife (age 45–55), not old age (over 65 or 75), images of menopause are confused with those of old age. The classic stereotype of a menopausal woman is highly negative: a wrinkled, stooped-over, and frail woman. Most women at age 50 do not have this appearance. However, in cultures that value youth and vitality, this association of menopause with aging influences the psychological impact of menopause (van Keep and Kellerhals 1974).

American society fosters excessive concern about youthfulness, healthiness, and wellness with the mandate that we should modify our behavior to ward off aging, illness, and death (Barsky and Klerman 1983). Because menopause is associated with aging, the emphasis on youth exerts pressure to eliminate or reverse the process of menopause. Some believe that we live in an overmedicalized culture that is obsessed with health and pathologically fearful of aging and death.

Socioeconomic Status and Ethnicity

For middle- and upper-class women, midlife may present many opportunities that were not available to them during the childbearing years. They may return to work and/or rewarding careers, travel and find other interests, and fully enjoy their postparental years. Studies have reported that women with less education (LaRocco and Polit 1980) and lower socioeconomic status (Jaszmann et al. 1969) have more symptoms at menopause. However, for some poor minority (primarily African American and Latina) women, the traumas of inner-city life may dwarf the changes of menopause. Other women must function as mothers for their grandchildren at this time as a result of working single mothers, poverty, and the urban substance abuse epidemic. (In Chapter 4 in this volume, Weber examines the cultural differences in menopause.)

Children Leaving Home

Traditionally, midlife was defined as the time when children left the home, but women now have children both earlier and later, so age and life phase may not correspond (Notman 1979). The "empty-nest syndrome" was proposed as a social cause of symptoms at menopause, but data indicate that this is a myth. The empty-nest syndrome is an outgrowth of the psychological loss theory, which posits that at menopause, a woman loses one of her major roles— that of mother—as well as the rewards that accompany it. Benedek (1950) predicted that women without children would have a more difficult time at menopause, but these women seem to confront this issue earlier and actually have an easier time at menopause (Notman 1979). Studies indicate that women who become depressed after their last child leaves home have been overinvolved with their children (Bart and Grossman 1978). In contrast, psychologically healthy women whose children have left home report greater happiness, life enjoyment, and marital satisfaction as compared with women at the same age who have at least one child living at home (Glenn 1975). Thus, a woman whose life is solely devoted to her children may feel useless and depressed when they leave, whereas a woman who has other sources of gratification, who is still married, and whose children live nearby and are a source of pleasure will likely have an easier time at midlife during the postparental phase.

Many women whose lives were restricted by the demands of child rearing welcome menopause and the new opportunities and freedom it provides. "Boomerang" adult children who return home may cause stress.

Case 1

Ms. A is 53 years old. She was working as a nurse when she met her successful businessman husband and left nursing to raise two sons, now 23 and 25 years old. Three months after her last menstrual period, she became depressed. Further investigation revealed that both sons had returned home after college, and the second son was still living at home, was not working, and had no plans for the future. Brief family therapy encouraged her son to develop a plan for a job search and independent living. Ms. A's mood improved, and she said, "I feel like I am the person I was. Before, I could only see the bad side. Now, I can see the bright side too." Ms. A was menopausal, but her problems were related not to menopause, but to the changes in her family coincidentally occurring at the same time.

Family Relationships

The menopausal years coincide with many stressful changes in the family. Teenaged and young adult children may be difficult to cope with and/or disappointing in terms of parental expectations. On the other hand, women who have not felt satisfied with their accomplishments might be envious of and compete with their children at this time of life. A common source of stress results from the woman's being caught between aging parents and dependent children, with those in this situation being referred to as the "sandwich generation." Parents and/or in-laws may be elderly and ailing, and women, more often than men, are recruited to care for elderly relatives at this time. Seventy-five percent of parents live within 30 minutes of one child, often turning to a daughter to help them with their concrete and emotional needs (Blume 1986).

Marital Issues

The effect of marital status on menopausal symptoms is not clear because good longitudinal data are not available. It may be the quality of the marital relationship that is significant rather than marital status per se. Separated, widowed, or divorced women seem to be at greatest risk for distress, followed by married women, with single women reporting the least depression (Avis and McKinlay 1995; Gove 1973; Hunter 1990; McKinlay et al. 1987). However, the higher socioeconomic status of women who never married confounds this finding. Health concerns of lesbian women are generally poorly described; thus, it is not surprising that no references were found about the lesbian experience of menopause.

Marital problems may arise from the midlife transition in men and the lack of synchrony in careers. A man may be at the peak or even the beginning of the decline of his career, whereas a woman who has taken time out for child rearing may be at an upwardly mobile time in her career. In addition, men may develop sexual problems at this time of life, which are caused by either psychological problems such as midlife crises or physical problems such as those related to medication, aging, or illness. This dysfunction can lead to extramarital affairs, marital disruption, and abandonment of wives. (See Lamont, Chapter 5, for a discussion of sexuality.)

Career and Work Issues

Working outside the home influences a woman's well-being at midlife and seems to be associated with fewer symptoms at menopause. Although stress is involved in trying to "have it all," studies indicate that assumption of multiple roles has a positive effect on physical and mental well-being (Barnett and Marshall 1991). Conversely, the scarcity hypothesis of the 1960s stated that people do not have enough energy to fulfill their role obligations, so the more roles one accumulates, the greater the probability of role strain and psychological distress (Goode 1960). The expansion hypothesis of the 1970s postulated that one's assuming multiple roles enhances well-being; this hypothesis has been supported by subsequent studies (Marks 1977). Research has suggested that it is not only working outside the home but also having a job in which one feels little satisfaction and has little control over the work, but the employer has a high level of demand, that is stressful. Therefore, it appears that working outside the home may actually buffer women from the stress associated with the maternal role (Wethington and Kessler 1989).

Social Context of Menopause

How society views menopause has a major effect on women's experience. Menopause has been conceptualized as both a nonadaptive and an adaptive event (Woods 1995). The nonadaptive conceptualization emphasizes generalized physiological decline and is consistent with medical intervention. A survey of primary care physicians found that 80% viewed menopause as an endocrine deficiency disease and saw women as vulnerable and at risk for disease (Woods 1995). This view reinforces a traditional notion of women as having value only as long as they have a childbearing function. When this function ends at menopause, women are depicted as being "over-the-hill," asexual, depressed, and debilitated. Women are bombarded by advertisements reminding them that now that they are living longer, they need treatment to keep their bodies young (Dickson 1995).

Conceptualizing menopause as an adaptive event for the species assumes that female humans have been selected to cease reproduction because there is a risk of reproduction in late life. This conceptualization suggests that older women may be of more use when they are available to rechannel their energies into caring for and supporting others, such as adult offspring and grandchildren. This conceptualization is consistent with the views of most midlife women who view themselves as healthy and free, mature, strong, resilient, and powerful. Women see themselves at the beginning of a new phase in their lives with relief from menses and reproductive responsibilities and freedom to try new options (Woods 1995).

Psychological Theories of Menopause

Historically, psychological theories about menopausal symptoms focused on the concept of loss and the symptoms of depression, assuming the same psychodynamics of depression for women as for men (Notman 1995). Modern theories about distress at menopause emphasize factors that are specific to women.

Loss of Connectedness

The new psychology of women has emphasized the increased importance of relationships and connectedness (Gilligan 1982; Miller 1993). Traditional psychological theory emphasized separation-individuation, which better characterizes the development of men, whereas the new psychology of women focuses on the value of relationships and connectedness. For example, "dependency" is viewed by traditional theorists as an immature stage to be overcome, but in the new psychology of women, it is viewed positively as a correlate of connectedness. Midlife changes and stresses often involve separations and distancing in relationships, which threaten a woman's sense of connectedness and may lead to distress.

Case 2

Ms. S was 51 years old when she was referred urgently by her husband's psychotherapist after a rare temper outburst at her difficult husband. The psychiatrist was urged to "do something" because Ms. S was "not herself" since her last menstrual period 5 months earlier. Investigation revealed that Ms. S's mother had died 1 year ago. Ms. S was overwhelmed with guilt. She had had little contact with her mother during childhood because of the mother's career, but they had been extremely close as adults. "My life stopped when my mother became ill." Ms. S was menopausal, but her problem was a pathological grief reaction, which responded to brief psychotherapy.

Loss of Self-Esteem

A stable sense of self is an important aspect of psychological health. Self-esteem is derived from not only experiences and relationships but also proper and effective functioning of one's body (Notman 1995). Women may feel inadequate when they do not feel good about their appearance or how it is regarded or if they are concerned about their sexual and reproductive functioning. Women with more symptoms at menopause have been found to have low self-esteem and low life satisfaction (R. J. Kraines: "The Menopause and Evaluations of the Self: A Study of Middle-Aged Women," unpublished doctoral dissertation, University of Chicago, Chicago, Illinois, 1963).

Loss of Reproductive Capacity

Classic psychoanalytic formulation assumed that women could not fulfill their sexual identity without having children and that menopause, with its loss of the capacity to reproduce, affected identity as a woman. Helene Deutsch reflected the dominant view of her time that femininity was defined by the possibility of pregnancy and that menopause was a "narcissistic mortification" that was "difficult to overcome." She wrote that a woman "loses all she received at puberty" and that mastery of menopause was one of the most difficult tasks of a woman's life. Deutsch saw increased activity postmenopause as a "struggle to preserve femininity" closely tied to sexual attractiveness and reproduction (Deutsch 1945). On the other hand, Theresa Benedek saw menopause as desexualizing emotional needs, releasing what Margaret Mead called post-menopausal zest (Benedek 1950).

Freud's idea that anatomy is destiny is true with regard to reproduction. The capacity to reproduce is one important aspect of feminine identity. Girls grow up assuming that they can carry and give birth to a baby. The time-limited nature of reproductive capacity influences a woman's life choices and her freedom to make them. Even if a woman does not plan to have a baby, the potential to bear children is part of her gender identity. Women who had hoped for children may be disappointed at the approach of menopause. For other women, even though they feel their family is complete, the loss of the capacity to reproduce may cause distress at menopause (Notman 1995).

Midlife as a Developmental Stage

In the new field of adult development, midlife is viewed as a phase in the life cycle representing the transition from early to late adulthood (Notman 1990); menopause is one of the midlife experiences of women. Traditionally, loss, including the loss of reproductive capacity, has been viewed negatively as an obstacle to be overcome, but it can also be conceptualized as a central element in development that is critical for growth. Because development requires a giving up and letting go of the past, loss can stimulate new development and new psychological organization (Notman 1990). For example, parents may view children's leaving home as a loss, but they might also view it as an extension and expansion of parenting to include wider interests and travel to places to visit their children (Notman 1990).

Midlife, as a developmental phase, is also characterized by separations and distancing in relationships. Examples are illness, divorce, death of a spouse, difficulties with teenaged or young adult children, issues of aging in parents or in-laws, and rejection by a society that idealizes youth and values men over women. Midlife has been compared to adolescence. Just as adolescents must separate from their parents and make their own way in the world, midlife women who may have been caring for children must separate from this role and from their children. This separation and distancing are difficult for women because the emphasis in women's development is on connectedness and relationships rather than on separation-individuation and work (Miller 1993). However, women at midlife have both the opportunity and the need to forge new meanings in their lives and develop their interests.

Midlife is characterized by the paradox of new opportunities as well as limitations. No wonder it may represent either a high or a low point in a woman's life. Menopause occurs at a time when many women are experiencing changes in roles, responsibilities, and relationships. This is also a time of increased reflection and introspection which, combined with the nonlinear timetable of women's development, may result in a time of increased energy and creativity. In fact, many women are relieved at the end of childbearing and have realistic opportunities to do things that were not possible during the childbearing years. Data from epidemiological studies indicate that natural menopause does not have a major negative effect on health or behavior (Avis and McKinlay 1995).

Psychologically, midlife is a phase when a person becomes aware that he or she has a finite amount of time left to live. The hopes and dreams of childhood and early adulthood are tempered by the reality of a limited perspective and limited possibilities, and women may be more vulnerable to loss at this time. These changes may create stress and affect identity, self-esteem, and social and family relationships (Matthews 1992).

Evolving Concepts of Menopause

Social forces in four periods—Victorian, psychoanalytic, biomedical, and "postmodern"—have influenced the scientific knowledge of menopause.

The Victorian medical view dominated social assumptions about menopause in the late nineteenth century. Women were warned that the hazards of menopause could be avoided if they held fast to their innate nurturing, delicate, and moral nature. Leeches and rest were prescribed.

The psychoanalytic view was dominant in the early to mid

twentieth century. Problems of menopause were seen as intrapsychic and caused by unresolved conflicts about being a woman.

The biomedical view or disease model, which followed the synthesis of estrogen in the 1930s, still dominates medicine today. In this model, menopause is viewed not as a life event but as an endocrinopathy requiring medical intervention and management. Although much has been written about the biopsychosocial model, medicine remains biomedically oriented, and psychosocial concerns are relatively ignored (Engel 1977; Notman 1995). The biomedical view or disease model is influenced by clinicians' experience in treating symptomatic menopausal women and is supported by studies of clinical populations. Both the psychoanalytic and the disease models tend to equate women with their reproductive systems and assume that when a woman can no longer reproduce, she is less of a woman.

The increase in the number of midlife women and increased freedom to speak about menopause have fostered the emergence of a new concept of menopause. The "postmodern" view followed the women's movement of the 1970s and is based on how women now view, experience, and gain knowledge about the menopausal transition (Dickson 1995). It emphasizes multiple sources of knowledge about menopause and the contribution of social, psychological, cultural, political, and economic variables as well as individual differences (Dickson 1995). Menopause is seen as a natural reproductive milestone in a woman's life, like menarche, rather than as an illness. Health promotion for midlife women is emphasized over the treatment of a hormone deficiency disease. In this view, the efficacy and safety of hormone use are considered important but as only one part of the scientific knowledge of menopause. Both the medical and the nonmedical views of menopause contain truth, but the lack of dialogue between them has created a dilemma for women.

Currently, most women neither see a physician nor take hormones for menopause (Oddens et al. 1992). Women are turning to self-help and are using a variety of remedies and support groups to facilitate harmonious aging, more like that of men. Recent popular books have helped to dispel the image of menopause as a dreaded time (Furman 1995).

Economic Factors

Economic forces in society foster the view of menopause as non-adaptive and requiring medical treatment. The 40 million menopausal women in the United States today create huge new markets for remedies, clinics, workshops, and books. In 1996, Premarin (conjugated estrogens tablets) was the most commonly prescribed drug in the United States, with prescriptions increasing by 10% a year (National Women's Health Resource Center, 2440 M Street, N.W., Suite 201, Washington, D.C., 20037, 1996 statistics).

Somatization

Midlife is characterized by many psychological and social sources of distress, and somatization is highly correlated with distress (Kellner 1990). Although the effect of stressful life events at midlife can be considerable and the relative contribution of menopause may be negligible, many women start to attribute symptoms to menopause during their 30s and 40s (Avis and McKinlay 1995).

A common presentation in menopause is acute situational stress such as frustration, disappointment, or loss associated with psychological and physical discomfort in the context of adjustment disorders (Sullivan and Katon 1993). Life change is correlated with the onset of psychological and physical disorders. As people become distressed, minor physical symptoms occur. Symptoms at menopause have been found to correlate with psychological and physical symptoms before menopause and negative attitudes toward menopause, as well as with the length of the perimenopause, lower educational level, and smoking (Avis and McKinlay 1995). Expectations about menopause can be related to symptom reporting, and negative attitudes can become a self-fulfilling prophecy (Avis and McKinlay 1995). Symptomatic treatment and reassurance usually are adequate to address these nonspecific symptoms, but menopausal women are often encouraged to take hormones.

Somatization is not an intrinsic property of the patient but is a pervasive process in medicine and results from the interaction of the patient with her sociocultural and medical environment. Physicians who view symptoms at menopause as caused by hormonal change may foster somatization and neglect treatable sources of psychosocial distress. The stigma of mental illness encourages patients to seek help for physical symptoms and deemphasize their depressive symptoms, which make the diagnosis difficult. Finally, factors that maintain or reinforce symptoms have been much better studied than those that initiate symptoms. Thus, the focus tends to be on the symptoms and their consequences rather than on midlife changes or stressors (Sullivan and Katon 1993).

Society holds patients accountable for psychological but not for physical distress, so physical symptoms can become a source of power for those who feel disenfranchised. Being sick can solve problems. Fortunately, in most cases, somatization is not severe and can be treated successfully by identifying the role that distress plays in symptom production and by reducing the distress (Sullivan and Katon 1993).

A Woman's Decision About Whether to Take Hormones

A woman's decision about whether or not to take hormones is based on how she views menopause as well as on biomedical considerations. Most women consider symptoms to be a natural part of menopause and feel that their symptoms are not severe enough to warrant medical consultation or hormone replacement. Of patients given hormone prescriptions, 25% do not fill them (Rowles 1990) and 50% do not continue taking them long term (Coope and March 1992). One-third of women who refuse hormones and one-third who stop taking them do so because of side effects, such as dysphoria or cyclic bleeding. For others, medication is associated with illness and disease, conditions that do not correspond to their experience of themselves at this time as being healthy. These women resist the implication that they have a deficiency disorder such as diabetes or hypothyroidism.

Women are also concerned that current data regarding the safety and efficacy of hormone use are inconclusive. Their fears of adverse consequences of taking hormones have been increased by the knowledge of previous bad outcomes with reproductive hormones such as diethylstilbestrol (DES) or the recently suggested association between hormones given for infertility treatment and development of ovarian cancer (Rossing et al. 1994). Twenty-five percent of women who refuse hormones and 20% of women who stop taking them do so for fear of breast cancer (Utian and Schiff 1994).

In the context of the medical and nonmedical view of menopause, poor communication with their physicians, societal pressure to stay young and healthy, and inadequate data, many women become preoccupied about whether to take hormones. Many women reluctantly decide to take hormones only after reading everything they can find and quizzing friends and experts. Some women who start taking hormones may be uncomfortable with their decision and so stop taking them.

Conclusion

The capacity to reproduce is not necessarily a dominating aspect of women's development, and loss of reproductive capacity need not be a central event in midlife or responsible for most midlife symptoms. To understand the psychosocial aspects of menopause, one must distinguish between menopause and the effects of aging and of midlife as a phase of adult development. To the extent that society devalues women and aging, menopause is seen as a problem rather than as a normal life transition. The dominance of the psychological loss theory of children leaving home was based on women being seen primarily as reproductive beings, but this theory appears to be outdated. In contrast, the new field of adult development views midlife as a developmental stage within the context of the new psychology of women and takes into account the differing timetables of women's development as compared with those of men. Poor communication between women and their physicians and neglect of psychosocial factors have hampered the understanding and alleviation of symptoms at menopause and may foster somatization.

References

Avis NE, McKinlay SM: The Massachusetts Women's Health Study: an epidemiologic investigation of the menopause. J Am Med Wom Assoc 50:45–49, 1995

Barnett RC, Marshall NL: Positive spillover effects from job to home: a closer look. Working Paper #222, Wellesley College Center for Research on Women, Wellesley, MA, 1991

Barsky AJ, Klerman GL: Overview: hypochondriasis, bodily complaints and somatic styles. Am J Psychiatry 140:273–283, 1983

Bart PB, Grossman M: Menopause, in The Woman Patient, Vol 1. Edited by Notman MT, Nadelson CC. New York, Plenum, 1978, pp 337–354

Benedek T: Climacterium: a developmental phase. Psychoanal Q 19:1–27, 1950

Blume SB: Women and alcohol. JAMA 256:1467–1470, 1986

Coope J, March J: Can we improve compliance with long-term HRT? Maturitas 15:151–158, 1992

Deutsch H: The Psychology of Women, Vol 1. New York, Grune & Stratton, 1945, pp 456–491

Dickson G: Paradigms of Menopause. Presented at a conference of the North American Menopause Society, San Francisco, CA, September 21–23, 1995

Engel GL: The need for a new medical model: a challenge for biomedicine. Science 196:129–136, 1977

Furman CS: The Myths and Realities of Menopause. New York, Oxford University Press, 1995

Gilligan C: Adult development and women's development: arrangements for a marriage, in Women in the Middle Years. Edited by Giele JZ. New York, Wiley, 1982, pp 89–114

Glenn ND: Psychological well-being in the post-parental stage: some evidence from national surveys. Journal of Marriage and the Family 32:105–110, 1975

Goode W: A theory of strain. American Sociological Review 25:483–496, 1960

Gove W: Sex, marital status and mobility. Am J Sociology 79:45–67, 1973

Hunter MS: Psychological and somatic experience of the menopause: a prospective study. Psychosom Med 52:357–367, 1990

Jaszmann L, VanLith ND, Zaat JCA: The perimenopausal symptoms: the statistical analysis of a survey. Medical Gynaecology and Sociology 4:268–277, 1969

Kellner R: Somatization: theories and research. J Nerv Ment Dis 178:150–160, 1990

LaRocco SA, Polit DF: Women's knowledge about the menopause. Nurs Res 29:10–13, 1980

Marks SR: Multiple roles and role strain: some notes on human energy, time and commitment. American Sociological Review 41:921–936, 1977

Matthews KA: Myths and realities of the menopause. Psychosom Med 54:1–9, 1992

McKinlay JB, McKinlay SM, Brambilla DJ: Health status and utilization behavior associated with menopause. Am J Epidemiol 125:110–121, 1987

Miller JB: A relational approach to understanding women's lives and problems. Psychiatric Annals 23:424–430, 1993

Notman M: Midlife concerns of women: implications of the menopause. Am J Psychiatry 136:1270–1274, 1979

Notman MT: Menopause and adult development. Multidisciplinary Perspectives on Menopause 592:149–155, 1990

Notman MT: Reproductive and critical transitions in the lifespan of women patients with focus on menopause. Depression 3:99–106, 1995

Oddens BJ, Boulet MS, Lehert P, et al: Has the climacteric been medicalized? A study on the use of medication for climacteric complaints in four countries. Maturitas 15:171–181, 1992

Rossing MA, Daling JR, Weiss NS, et al: Ovarian tumors in a cohort of infertile women. N Engl J Med 331:771–776, 1994

Rowles TB: Third International Symposium on Osteoporosis and Consensus Development Conference, Copenhagen, 1990. Copenhagen, Osteopress, 1990

Schmidt PJ, Rubinow DR: Menopause-related affective disorders: a justification for further study. Am J Psychiatry 148:884–852, 1991

Sullivan M, Katon W: Somatization: the path between distress and somatic symptoms. American Pain Society Journal 2:141–149, 1993

Utian WH, Schiff I: NAMS—Gallup survey on women's knowledge, information sources and attitudes to menopause and hormone replacement therapy. Menopause 1:39–48, 1994

van Keep PA, Kellerhalls JM: The impact of socio-cultural factors on symptom formation. Psychother Psychosom 23:251–263, 1974

Wethington E, Kessler RC: Employment, parental responsibility and psychological distress: a longitudinal study of married women. Journal of Family Issues 10:527–546, 1989

Woods NF: Menopause, Models, Medicine and Midlife. Presented at a conference of the North American Menopause Society, San Francisco, CA, September 21–23, 1995

CHAPTER 4

Cross-Cultural Menopause: A Study in Contrasts

Gail G. Weber, B.Sc.N., M.Sc.

The story goes . . .

> There is an indigenous tribe that lives in a far off land where it is believed that women will die once their menstrual periods stop. In this far off land, women do not experience menopause until they are in their eightieth year.

Variations on this fable are heard every now and then at meetings and conferences where professionals gather to discuss cross-cultural studies and/or menopause. Sadly, nobody has observed this unique society, and no references to it are found in the anthropological literature. Nonetheless, this story is important because it speaks of the power of a cultural belief system and the importance of a community of support; these elements are essential in the understanding of cross-cultural phenomena (Northrup 1994).

Introduction:
The Cultural Construction of Menopause

If menopause were simply a biological event, we could then assume a certain universality of experience cross-culturally. Instead, we find that the only universal truths about menopause are that it is decidedly a female experience and that it marks the end of menstruation and fertility. But beyond this, its meanings, its physical manifestations, and the social changes it produces vary greatly from culture to culture. As with menarche, pregnancy, and childbirth, the experience of menopause is deeply embedded within the context of women's lives. Menopause is not "a thing unto itself"; it is shaped, defined, and constructed by the culture in which it takes place.

In this chapter, I examine the experience of menopause in midlife women from a cross-cultural perspective, looking specifically at the subjective symptomatology reported by women and the "change of life" that menopause may herald for them. In addition, I examine some of the theoretical speculations about the role of biology, culture, and aging in the menopause. I describe a cross-cultural assessment tool and make some recommendations that health care professionals may find helpful in their interactions with middle-aged women from diverse cultures.

A cross-cultural analysis must provide a broad perspective on the experience and interpretation of menopause, and it must challenge us to reexamine our own cultural beliefs. By investigating various explanatory models other than the biomedical paradigm, it quickly becomes apparent that the biomedical model of menopause, in itself, neglects the existence of a social or cultural context in women's lives.

Menopause in North America

Much of the research to date on menopause has been done with Caucasian women in North America and Europe (Lock et al. 1988). A stereotypical picture of the perimenopausal woman has been extrapolated from these research studies, which are usually based on clinical rather than general population samples (Kaufert 1982). (This methodological issue is also discussed in Chapters 6, 7, 8, 9, and 10.) As a result of many clinical studies, researchers have assumed that the findings are true for all women universally, across culture, ethnicity, race, and socioeconomic class.

In North America, a commonly anticipated depiction of a menopausal woman is that of a depressed woman who is grieving the loss of her youth, her beauty, her sexuality, her power, and her mothering role (see Gise, Chapter 3, and Lamont, Chapter 5, in this volume). Typically, this menopausal woman is clinically reported as presenting with hot flashes, night sweats, vaginal dryness, insomnia, mood swings, and depression. In addition, the postmenopausal woman is considered to be at dire risk for osteoporosis and heart disease, as well as other deteriorating diseases related to aging (see Mogul, Chapter 6, in this volume). This characterization tends to form an archetype of the menopausal woman that then defines in our minds the anticipated menopausal experience of women in North America (see Chapter 6).

The biomedical model characterizes menopause as "ovarian failure" or as an "estrogen deficiency disease" (Wilson 1966). Therefore, if menopause is defined as an "organ failure," then the physician is obliged to provide treatment (see Shapiro, Chapter 7, in this volume). Despite this "medicalization" of menopause, it is interesting to note that the portrayal of the archetypal menopausal woman does not conform well to the actual and lived experience of most North American women. Yet, the mythology of menopausal distress continues to cast its shadow on women's anticipation of menopause. Lock and Kaufert (1992) found that the experiences of North American women were often in contrast to the archetypal Westernized picture of menopausal women. Certainly, in the West, the classic symptoms of hot flashes and night sweats were reported frequently, but many women also viewed menopause as a time of good health, new opportunities, and vigor, and they did not anticipate major difficulties. This discrepancy between the medical literature's portrayal of menopausal women and the way in which women actually experience menopause adds to the confusion about menopause in North America (Beyene 1989; Griffin 1977).

One aspect of menopause that North American women must deal with and that, as yet, is not part of the experience of most Third World women is the use or nonuse of hormone replacement therapy. North American women often experience considerable anxiety in regard to decision making about hormone use because much of the medical information about its safety is contradictory. In fact, the anxiety involved in this decision may accentuate the difficulty some women have and identify as associated with menopause.

Cross-Cultural Menopause

Investigators find that few of the "typical symptoms," or the psychosocial characterization of middle-aged women, hold true cross-culturally. In many cultures, menopause usually is not defined as anything but a normal, natural part of aging. The reporting of problematic symptoms varies among cultures and may, in fact, be absent or much less frequent among non-Western, nonindustrialized cultures than among Western cultures (Brown 1992). Symptoms, if present, may be "atypical," or they may have different meanings (Skultans 1970).

Menopause and Midlife: A Social Context

In examining some of the classic anthropological studies of menopause and of midlife in women, researchers recognize that they are indeed dealing with studies in contrast, not only in terms of menopause but also in relation to the social status, the roles, and the prestige that women hold in their middle years. Menopause cannot be separated from the social context of midlife and aging and the social positions that women hold in their later years (see Chapter 3).

Status change in midlife is, in many ways, paradoxical. For example, in many Third World countries, women are valued in their later years and are greatly restricted during adolescence and young adulthood. Conversely, in North America, women have more power and social status as young adults, and these characteristics decline sharply as women age (Bart 1969). In both cultures, to a large degree, women's position in life is still, and sadly too often, determined by their reproductive abilities and/or sexual attractiveness. Bart (1969) found that, in general, a woman's position in society increased in later life when the following factors were present: reversal of strong menstrual taboos, an extended family system as opposed to a nuclear family system, age valued more than youth, reproduction valued more than sexuality, close maternal-child relationships in later life, and institutionalized roles for grandmothers and mothers-in-law.

Positive changes in the lives of middle-aged women in many cultures result primarily from the withdrawal of restrictions based on menstrual and sexual taboos. Once these taboos are lifted, women become part of a highly respected senior generation. They can then interact informally with men, have more geographic mobility, and have special status in the community. As senior persons in the extended family network, middle-aged women have authority over and respect from their daughters and daughters-in-law. In addition, they have the support given by adult children (including their sons and sons-in-law), all of which is "so central to the definition of middle aged women cross culturally and so crucial to their relatively privileged position" (Brown 1992, p. 21).

Correlations between increased status and the lack of menopausal symptoms have been suggested as an explanation for differences in the menopausal experience (Flint 1975). Flint suggested that the difficulties with menopause experienced by some North American women may be related to the decline in social status and prestige that comes with aging in Western culture. Thus, social factors such as low self-esteem and internalized negative attitudes toward aging, not just fluctuating hormones, conceivably may be involved in menopausal distress (Flint 1975).

Cross-Cultural Social Implications of Menopause

Flint's (1975) study of Rajput Indian women found that menopause was not associated with problematic symptoms of hot flashes, night sweats, or depression. In fact, the cessation of menses was the only change reported. For these women, menopause resulted in a positive role change because they were now able to leave their veiled seclusion and become part of the larger community. Flint's work suggests an association between a positive role change and the lack of menopausal problems.

In a small study of midlife Welsh women, Skultans (1970) reported that although the women studied did experience hot flashes, they welcomed them as signs of a quick and healthy journey through menopause. This is an excellent example of the cultural reframing of a negative event into a more positive experience, not unlike the redesignation by modern American feminists of the hot flash into a "surge of power."

Lee's (1992) study of !Kung women of Botswana, South Africa, found that "the status of !Kung women, generally high, increases with age and reaches a peak in the decades after the childbearing tasks are completed. The postmenopausal !Kung woman is a mover and shaker in !Kung society" (p. 36). He noted that life is less burdensome for older women in this culture because they are relieved of many childbearing and household tasks. Lee pointed out that "the !Kung, in common with other third world women, undergo a blossoming rather than a shrinking or contraction [in midlife]" (p. 43).

The term *Tamparonga, "The Big Women,"* is an expression of honor and respect for older women among the Lusi people of Papua, New Guinea (Ayers Count 1992). The word *tamparonga* itself refers to a female elder (Ayers Count 1992). Lusi women become "Big Women" when they have grandchildren and are themselves near the end of childbearing. No word exists in the Lusi language for middle age or for menopause, and menopause apparently has no special significance for them. In my study of five ethnocultural communities in Toronto, Ontario (Weber 1994), I observed that the term *Big Woman* was also used as a term of respect and honor for older women in both the Somalian and the Caribbean communities.

Social Implications of Menopause in North America

The contrast in terms of status between the life of a stereotypical Westernized woman and women in the other cultures described above is often striking. Particularly in North American culture, the middle-aged woman may, in some cases, be living alone, be divorced or widowed, and have few family or social supports. Her children do not just leave the nest; they often move across the country, because the labor market, rather than family, seems to dictate life choices. Relationships with adult children are often reduced to occasional visits, obligatory telephone calls, letters, and brief holiday visits. The role of mother-in-law, rather than being respected and honored, is, all too often, the butt of jokes, and she is usually characterized as bossy and intrusive. Generally, midlife and older women in North America are poorer, have far fewer opportunities in the job market, and need more social supports than do most other groups.

Nonetheless, midlife women now are increasingly realizing that the freedom from family and household responsibilities does present new choices and opportunities. Although first-time job opportunities may be difficult to find, increasing numbers of women older than 45 years are returning to work, to school, and to the community, where their skills can be well utilized and appreciated. Despite these significant advances, however, women often experience these middle years as a time of considerable loss. Because there are no predetermined and honored roles that middle-aged women in North American society can assume with ease, they must often struggle to redefine new roles and new images of the self. To accomplish this, they must negotiate in a world that may be indifferent and even hostile to older women. These circumstances certainly present a more difficult context in which to experience menopause than that of middle-aged women whose social status increases with age.

A significant question emerges: Just how much does the social context in which a woman lives affect the menopausal experience? If, as Flint (1975) suggested, there is a correlation between a woman's social position in midlife and menopausal symptoms, then it is understandable why menopause may be difficult for some North American women and why these women and their physicians may view menopause as a disease. The emphasis on youth, beauty, and fertility in Western culture may make the menopause, or reconstruct it into, a difficult experience. Fears about being alone and being out of the mainstream of life are part of the anxiety experienced by middle-aged women in North America. In fact, fears about aging usually far outweigh concerns about hot flashes or vaginal dryness.

The Need for a Multivariant Analysis

Feminists have often been critical of the biomedical model, when used as the sole observational platform, because it tends to draw linear-causal relationships between a decrease in estrogen and an array of menopausal symptoms, and it often generates dire health predictions. By the same token, it is imperative to avoid drawing the same sort of facile analysis with linear-causal depictions of the relationship between lowered social status and the existence of problematic symptoms. Context is essential to a feminist analysis, and the context must include a multiplicity of variables, both socio-cultural and biological.

North American society, like most cultures, is in transition to some degree. Fifty years ago, we did not anticipate sociocultural changes in our lives such as increased divorce rates, the massive reentry of women into the job market, or the rise of professional life among women. Nor could we anticipate the emergence of the women's movement and feminism and the changes these efforts would bring about. These recent and major social changes have had profound influences on women's lives. Mostly anecdotal in-formation has informed us about how these social transitions have affected women's experience of menopause. We have not yet ex-amined the effect of socioeconomic class, race, ethnicity, religion, and marginalization on the menopause. Unfortunately, as long as we continue to rely solely on a biomedical model for explanations of menopause, we will miss the opportunity to examine the effects of some of these social changes and transitions on women's meno-pause experience within American culture.

The work of Yewoubdar Beyene and Margaret Lock has added greatly to the understanding of the sociocultural and biological fac-tors involved in menopause. They have added to the anthropologi-cal analysis of menopause by including in their inquiry factors such as diet, fertility patterns, lactational activity, physical activity, and genetic influences as well as sociocultural considerations.

A Study of Two Peasant Cultures: Mayan and Greek

Beyene (1989) set out to examine the social environment of older women in two peasant cultures—one Mayan and one Greek—to determine how social context influences menopause. She found similar values and belief systems in both cultures; also, midlife and older women had expanded roles and increased social status. In addition, both cultures had strong menstrual taboos wherein women were considered unclean and contaminated during menstruation, thus limiting their participation in community and religious life. With their entry into menopause, both communities of women were freed from taboos and restrictions and were able to enjoy more religious, community, and sexual freedoms. In both cultures, middle-aged women held positions of authority as heads of extended family households. Old age was associated with increased power, respect, and status for these women, especially when their sons married. The sociocultural environments of the two societies are similar and certainly positive in terms of role and status change. And yet, the experience of menopause itself is decidedly different for Mayan and for Greek peasant women.

For Mayan women, menopause is not associated with any physical or emotional changes. Cessation of menstruation is the only change reported, and menopause is welcomed. There are no reports of hot flashes, night sweats, or anxiety. Menopause is not viewed as a negative event, and the women report that they feel "free like a young girl again" and are "content and in good health" (Beyene 1989, p. 130).

In contrast, the menopause experience of the rural Greek women is more typical of that of women in Western industrialized cultures. They experience hot flashes, night sweats, and a variety of other physical difficulties. They perceive menopause negatively and have anxiety and concern about future health problems. They have fears about growing older, despite the increased status they have achieved with age. Even though Greek women have hot flashes, they do not perceive them as disease and generally do not seek medical treatment for them. They see hot flashes as a natural phenomenon causing temporary discomfort.

In this comparison, Beyene hypothesized that "the existence or the lack of physiological symptoms cannot be explained in terms of role change in midlife or by the removal of cultural taboos" (p. 131). Other factors must be involved to account for the differences in the experiences of women in these two cultures. She suggested that differences in fertility patterns, lactational patterns, and diet may, in fact, affect the production of estrogen and thus result in certain physiological changes.

Fertility Patterns Among
Mayan and Greek Peasant Women

Mayan women do not use birth control and have many pregnancies. In addition, with prolonged breast-feeding, they may not have steady or regular menstrual periods for most of their reproductive lives. This pattern is fairly typical of many Third World cultures where fertility patterns may be such that it is not uncommon for a woman to experience up to 15 years of amenorrhea due to pregnancy and breast-feeding and to have only about 4 years of menstruation during the entire reproductive life cycle (Konner and Worthman 1980).

In contrast, Greek women use birth control and have few pregnancies, with planned family size. They breast-feed for shorter periods and have more regular and more frequent menstruation. Estrogen production is likely affected by differences in these fertility patterns. Similarly, it has been suggested that for women in more industrialized and Westernized countries, "decreased childbearing with short periods of lactational postpartum amenorrhea possibly exposes the body to more estrogen stimulation and its sudden decline could be manifested in both hot flashes and bone density loss" (Beyene 1989, p. 137).

Dietary Considerations Among
Mayan and Greek Peasant Women

The ecology of both regions studied is different, which results in differences in dietary composition. The diet of the Mayan women primarily consists of corn, beans, tomatoes, and camote (sweet potatoes). These people have very little animal protein in their diet and virtually no milk products. The diet of the Greek women includes a wider variety of foods, with wheat, cheese, milk, eggs, olives, and legumes. There is plenty of meat, fish, fruit, and wine. Variations in hormone production between different populations may partly be accounted for by differences in diet, because diet is thought to affect both ovarian function and adrenal activity (MacMahon et al. 1974).

Physical Activity, Diet, and Osteoporosis Among Mayan and Greek Peasant Women

In both cultures, osteoporosis is not seen as a problem (Beyene 1989), and it may well be that high levels of physical activity and diet protect older women from osteoporotic fractures. Although large-scale cross-cultural studies of rates of osteoporosis have not been done, one study of the prevalence of osteoporotic fractures in nonindustrialized cultures indicated that they were rare (Nordin 1966). Current assumptions that indicate a direct linear relationship between menopause and osteoporosis are challenged by some cross-cultural studies, which indicate that "hormonal factors do not seem to explain all the variation in risk of postmenopausal osteoporotic fractures across racial and ethnic groups" (Beyene 1989, p. 24).

Beyene's work adds important facets to the study of menopause cross-culturally. Her findings suggest that factors such as status gain and the removal of menstrual taboos are inadequate explanations for cross-cultural variation and that it is essential to include other factors such as fertility patterns, physical activity, and diet.

Menopause in Japan

Lock's (1986) study of menopause in modern-day Japan provides further insight into "the cultural construction of menopause." Japan is a highly industrialized, technological society, not unlike American society with respect to modernity. However, the experience of menopause for Japanese women is remarkably different from that of American women.

Japanese women, unlike the North American woman with the stereotypical presentation, report few menopausal symptoms, and the symptoms they do report are different from those that are thought to be typical of a decrease in estrogen production. The classic hot flash, so often seen as the one "true" symptom of menopause, is reported so infrequently that no Japanese word exists to describe the hot flash. Night sweats, anxiety, and depression are also rarely reported by Japanese women. Instead, the symptoms reported, if at all, tend to be those of shoulder stiffness, headaches, backaches, and lack of energy. In addition, cardiovascular disease and osteoporosis are not frequently diagnosed among Japanese women. In general, menopause is seen as a natural life transition, a biological marker, but one that is not of great significance in life. It is simply considered as part of the more inclusive experience of *konenki,* a transitional stage of age. Konenki is associated with many life changes of aging, including a period of freedom from family responsibilities, and, as such, it is a welcomed period of life.

Life for modern Japanese women is, in many ways, a mixture of a traditional lifestyle with the beginnings of more Westernized influences. Despite much postwar social change in Japan, and despite an increase in Western influences, divorce is rare, age is respected, and most older people still prefer to live with their children. Embedded in Japanese philosophy is the belief in harmony between one's social and physical environment, and, to a great extent, there are supportive structures in society to help achieve this balance. Traditionally, the position of the older Japanese woman was an honored one, in which she reigned supreme over the extended household, with deference from her children and the ability to delegate responsibilities. Some current social changes have not been to her advantage, however. Although changes are occurring slowly in the extended family structure, it is apparent that the nuclear family arrangement is becoming increasingly evident. The middle-aged Japanese woman may now find herself, like her North American sisters, in an empty apartment with little to do. Menopause, in Japan, has been referred to as a "luxury disease for those with idle hands." The implicit expectation is that a Japanese woman should put the needs of the family and especially elderly family members ahead of her own needs. The expectation is also that she should go through menopause without complaint.

Dietary and Other Factors Affecting Menopause in Japan

The fact that Japanese women do not seem to experience physiological changes such as the hot flash may perhaps be understood by examining factors that affect biological change. The Japanese diet may provide some clues because it not only is low in fat and animal protein but also contains many foods with phytoestrogens (plants containing estrogen), such as tofu, green beans, alfalfa, flax-seed oils, and rice. Miso soup and many soy products, which are also part of the Japanese diet, contain phytoestrogens. Comparisons of the dietary patterns of Japanese women and Caucasian women show that different populations of comparable age may, in fact, have different plasma levels of hormones. Dietary factors such as fat intake and body weight may influence hormonal profiles in women (Hill 1977). In addition, genetic factors may help to explain the absence of hot flashes and other physiological changes thought to be caused by decreased estrogen.

Implications of a Multicultural Population

Increasingly, in North America, there is recognition of cultural diversity. With steady increases in immigration, health care practitioners must be sensitive to people who may experience health and illness differently.

Sensitivity to the Experiences of Culture and Immigration

The experience of immigration itself is a stressful one that involves many significant losses. As S. Blacker (unpublished manuscript, February 1995) points out, "Women who have immigrated to a culture that perceives physiological changes differently from their own understanding may find themselves confused when presented with treatments that do not meet their needs or address their real problems." The following case example offers an opportunity to consider the multifaceted nature of cross-cultural menopause practice:

Case Example

Ms. J, a 53-year-old woman, recently immigrated to the United States from the Caribbean. She left behind her husband, grown children, and grandchildren in the hope that she would find work and that they would join her in America. She began experiencing insomnia, fatigue, and feelings of depression and was seen by a family physician in a clinic. Because she is menopausal, the physician assumed that her depression was hormonally based and prescribed hormone replacement therapy. Unfortunately, hormone replacement therapy is not appropriate therapy for depression. In addition, the distress she experienced was largely the result of loneliness and the ageism and racism she was finding in the job market. This type of situational depression does not respond to hormone replacement therapy either. By solely focusing on Ms. J's biological functioning and neglecting the other aspects of her life, the physician may well have missed the opportunity to deal with the true source of her distress.

Practical Strategies for Working With Women From Diverse Cultures

An assessment tool that can be easily used with a patient is presented in Figure 4–1. It will assist the health care provider in exploring with the woman the sociocultural and biological context of her menopause.

Some Suggestions for Improving Cross-Cultural Communication

In general, it is best not to assume that menopause is a problem for women of other cultures. In many cultures, menopause is not seen as a source of difficulty. Instead, the clinician should use the following suggestions:

1. Find out from the patient about her experiences and knowledge of menopause. What does she think happens at menopause, and what does she anticipate?
2. Discuss the importance of a healthy diet and physical exercise with her. Be aware that food and even activity are culturally specific.
3. Have written materials (and audiovisual materials if possible) available that discuss menopause from a culturally relevant health promotion and lifestyle perspective. These materials should deal with information gathering, stress, exercise, social supports, and nutrition.

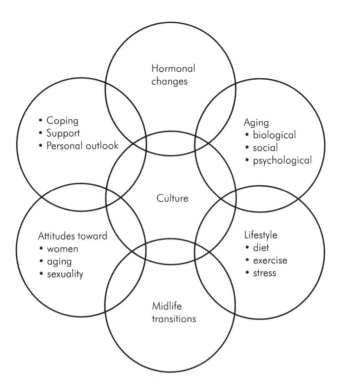

Figure 4–1. Context of menopause: a cross-cultural perspective illustrates the interactive and contextual nature of menopause. This tool can be used to discuss with a woman the various factors that may influence her menopausal experience. "Culture is placed in the middle because it is the factor that informs or shapes all others" (S. Blacker, unpublished manuscript, February 1995). This approach allows women to speak of their own experiences as they have been formed by their culture, their race, or their class. Designed by Gail Weber (1991). Adapted by Susan Blacker (1995), Women's College Hospital, Toronto, Canada.

4. Find out whether information and educational materials are available in different languages, and, if possible, have these accessible.

5. Be aware of community resources in women's health and in the ethnocultural communities, and refer for counseling and/or groups when appropriate. Also, be aware of the availability of interpreter and translator services if needed.

6. Recognize that in many cultures, menopause, women's bodies, and sexuality are difficult issues for women to discuss, so it is important to be available to listen but also to be respectful of silence.
7. Be prepared to discuss and explain issues of choice in terms of menopause treatment. It is important not only to discuss pros and cons of treatment but also to be clear that it is a woman's decision as to whether she will undergo treatment.
8. Be aware that courses and seminars are increasingly available for health professionals to learn cross-cultural communication, counseling skills, and sensitivity.
9. Realize that many different ethnocultural groups have made their homes in North America. It has been said that in the greater Los Angeles area alone, more than 120 different languages are spoken. This finding probably holds true for almost all major American cities today. We cannot learn all of these languages, but we can be aware of resources that may be helpful to the women with whom we are working. An enormous number of ethnically diverse groups compose American cities today. We cannot begin to describe their particular views on health, menopause, aging, or anything else. Nor do I think it serves us well to list ethnic characteristics and attitudes. Although large population groups of African Americans, Latinos, Chinese, Japanese, South Asians, Native Americans, and dozens more live in North America, it is imperative for us to recognize the enormous diversity that exists within these cultures. This intracultural diversity is based on socioeconomic class, geography, generational cohort, gender, degree of acculturation, language skills, age, occupation, and, most significantly, the length of time in North America.

Having said this, some generalizations can be made, and some basic principles may be useful in dealing with patients from other countries. For many of the ethnocultural communities, family is often extended and of primary importance. Family members may need to be involved in decisions about health and health care because interdependence with kin is often important. Respect for elders and for authority may also be an important value for many ethnocultural groups. In addition, in many cultures, there may be knowledge of, and respect for the use of, nontraditional or alternative medicine. It would be helpful for health care providers to be open to, and respectful of, other ways of healing. Basically, we communicate our warmth and caring in a nonverbal way; thus, we can be comfortable with our communication if we are sincere in our dealings with people.

The Future

Continued research into the menopausal experience of women from different ethnocultural backgrounds is necessary. African American women, Hispanic women, Asian women, and others can inform us about their views and experiences of menopause. In addition, longitudinal studies of women who were born in other countries and are now living in North America (Canada and the United States) must be developed to determine how different cultural practices may change over time and ultimately affect menopause. Further cross-cultural research is also needed in the areas of nutrition, physical activity, fertility patterns, and genetic differences, as well as in the psychosocial aspects of life. There is also much to learn from women of other cultures in terms of ancestral ways of dealing with the menopause and traditional ways of staying in good health. Margaret Lock, a medical anthropologist, spoke at the 1995 meeting of the North American Menopause Society in San Francisco, noting that "findings from Japan and other societies with similarly low symptom reporting suggest that it would be expedient to carry out future research designed to reveal what factors protect certain women from menopausal symptoms." These are challenging and complex questions that we should direct some research dollars toward investigating.

References

Ayers Count D: Tamparonga "The big women" of Kaliai, in In Her Prime: New Views of Middle Aged Women, 2nd Edition. Edited by Kerns V, Brown JK. Chicago, University of Illinois Press, 1992, pp 61–74

Bart P: Why women's status changes in middle age: the turns of the social ferris wheel. Sociological Symposium 3:1–18, 1969

Beyene Y: From Menarche to Menopause: Reproductive Lives of Peasant Women in Two Cultures. Albany, State University of New York Press, 1989

Brown JK: Lives of middle aged women, in In Her Prime: New Views of Middle Aged Women, 2nd Edition. Edited by Kerns V, Brown JK. Chicago, University of Illinois Press, 1992, pp 17–30

Flint M: The menopause: reward or punishment? Psychosomatics 16:161–163, 1975

Griffin JA: A cross cultural investigation of behavioural changes at menopause. The Social Science Journal 14:49–55, 1977

Hill P: Diet and endocrine-related cancer. Cancer 39:1820–1826, 1977

Kaufert P: Anthropology and the menopause: the development of a theoretical framework. Maturitas 4:181–193, 1982

Konner M, Worthman C: Nursing frequency, gonadal function and birth spacing among !Kung hunters/gathers. Science 207:788–791, 1980

Lee RB: Work, sexuality, and aging among !Kung women, in In Her Prime: New Views of Middle Aged Women, 2nd Edition. Edited by Kerns V, Brown JK. Chicago, University of Illinois Press, 1992, pp 35–44

Lock M: Ambiguities of aging: the Japanese experience and perceptions of menopause. Cult Med Psychiatry 10:23–46, 1986

Lock M, Kaufert P: "What are women for?" Cultural construction of menopausal women in Japan and Canada, in In Her Prime: New Views of Middle Aged Women, 2nd Edition. Edited by Kerns V, Brown JK. Chicago, University of Illinois Press, 1992, pp 201–219

Lock M, Kaufert P, Gilbert P: Cultural construction of the menopause syndrome: the Japanese case. Maturitas 10:317–322, 1988

MacMahon B, et al: Urine estrogen profiles of Asian and North American women. Int J Cancer 14:161–167, 1974

Nordin C: International patterns of osteoporosis. Clin Orthop 45:17–30, 1966

Northrup C: An M.D. speculates on menopause possibilities: interviewed by Judith S. Askew. Menopause News 4:1–4, 1994

Skultans V: The symbolic significance of menstruation and the menopause. Manushi: A Journal About Women and Society 5:639–651, 1970

Weber G: Celebrating Women, Aging and Cultural Diversity. Toronto, Ontario, Stand Alone Productions, 1994

Wilson RA: Feminine Forever. New York, M Evans, 1966

Sexuality

John A. Lamont, M.Sc., M.D., F.R.C.S.C.

Cultural context defines women's roles (see Weber, Chapter 4, in this volume). In some societies, including North American, a woman's procreative potential is an important and valued asset. In this context, a woman's worth may be determined by fecundity and attractiveness, whereas menopause may herald the end of the useful life and the loss of femininity, attractiveness, mental stability, and sexuality (Roughan et al. 1993). An opposing view has evolved over the last quarter century as women have struggled for equality, and some groups view menopause as a nonevent (see Stewart and Robinson, Chapter 1, in this volume). A woman's transition through the perimenopause is also influenced by intrapsychic and relationship factors (see also Gise, Chapter 3, in this volume). A sense of competence in a variety of roles, strong social and family supports, and financial security are positive factors in a woman's adaptation to change. Most women live through the menopausal transition without difficulty and continue to enjoy fulfilling sexual lives. However, women who face this transition alone, or see their role solely as procreant, will likely experience more physical, psychological, and sexual difficulties (Psarakis et al. 1990).

Physiological Changes Related to Sexual Function

Physiological sexual changes with aging have been well documented by Masters and Johnson (1966) (Table 5–1). These changes

Table 5–1. Normal age-related changes in sexual response in women

Arousal
Decreased elasticity of the vagina (foreshortening)
Decreased volume and speed of vaginal lubrication
Decreased and slower vaginal expansion

Orgasm
Fewer orgasmic contractions

Extragenital
Less intense "sex flush"
Reduced breast enlargement with arousal
Less intense anal sphincter contraction

Other
Postcoital vaginal irritation
Postcoital dysuria and urgency

can be summarized as decreased intensity of physiological response and decreased rapidity of sexual response in both men and women. Hormonal changes at menopause result in a dramatic decrease in estradiol production. Estradiol's effects on pelvic tissues to enhance sexual function are increased blood flow to the vulva and vagina as well as maintenance of the health of the vaginal epithelium for coital function (McCoy et al. 1985; Semmens and Wagner 1982).

The most common clinical symptom affecting sexual activity after menopause is dyspareunia. This symptom is often secondary to atrophy of the vaginal mucosa with loss of estradiol production from the ovary (see also Baram, Chapter 2, in this volume). Other estrogen-dependent changes in the vagina are a decline in the speed and volume of vaginal lubrication and a foreshortening of the vagina with age. If these difficulties are not corrected and attempts at coitus continue, the woman may develop a secondary vaginismus as a result of continued pain. The vaginismus then becomes a third factor contributing to her discomfort. Because the urethra and trigone are estrogen sensitive, some women develop 1 or 2 days of postcoital dysuria (Lamont 1994). Women may also have occasional stress incontinence, including incontinence during coital thrusting.

Hormonal influence on female mammals and human sexual behavior has been identified for more than 50 years. Beach (1976) suggested that sexual attractiveness and receptivity are controlled by estrogen, but proceptive behavior is augmented by androgens. The effect of androgens on sexual appetite in humans has been reported since 1941 (Greenblatt et al. 1942). Despite this, the influence of sex hormones on libido and sexual function is not clear. Research shows that sexual interest and capacity for sexual response are not entirely dependent on estrogen (Bachmann 1993).

Androgens appear to play some role in female sexual function. They are important for the development of female sexuality, but societal and peer influences all play critical roles (Bancroft 1987). Despite Kaplan and Owett's (1993) description of "The Female Androgen Deficiency Syndrome," there is no clear-cut relationship between circulating androgen level and sexual desire or frequency of sexual activity. Women with above-average levels of testosterone may have subjective and objective evidence of increased arousability (Lamont and Leitch 1995).

Women who undergo natural menopause retain some degree of androgen production from residual stromal cells of the ovary. Women who have surgical menopause experience a sudden, dramatic loss of both estradiol and ovarian androgens. These two sex steroids affect the dopaminergic and serotonergic neurotransmitter systems implicated in sexual behavior (Sherwin 1992). Both neurotransmitters appear to affect portions of the brain that are thought to subserve emotion and sexuality in humans.

Studies of hormone replacement show that estrogen replacement increases vaginal lubrication, blood supply, and expansion. Some studies of sexual interest during hormone replacement show no effect or improvement by estrogen, by androgens, or by both (Bancroft 1987).

Sexuality and Aging

The perimenopausal transition is physiological evidence of aging (see also Feldman and Netz, Chapter 12, in this volume). The physiological changes that accompany aging in women have not been shown to impair enjoyment of physical intimacy or the experience of sexual desire, arousal, or orgasm. Although women are more likely than men to report an improvement in sex over a lifetime (Winn and Newton 1982), most studies suggest a decline in sexual function with age when function equates sexual activity with frequency of intercourse. Studies of all sexual activity with aging reveal a surprisingly high prevalence of interest, arousal, and function.

The effect of aging on sexuality is also influenced by sociocultural beliefs and attitudes. In a society such as North America, where youth and beauty are equated with sexuality, there are many barriers to sexual expression (Lamont 1994). Data that are available with respect to traditional societies (i.e., native people of all countries) indicate that the majority of societies report the continuance of various kinds of sexual activity with aging (70% for men and 84% for women) (Kligman 1991). This literature also suggests that the level of sexual interest and activity is greater in women than in men. The majority (82%) of studies found that older women had much younger men as sexual partners. In cultures in which the major role of women is procreation, a decline in sexual activity of older women was noted.

Prevalence of Change in Sexual Function

Changes in physiological sexual response are inevitable with advancing years in both men and women. Pfeiffer and Davis (1972) found that 40% of women older than 60 years continued to engage in coital activity. In this study, a woman's sexual activity was found to be secondary to and dependent on a man's sexual desire and ability to function. Despite this, 13% of the women in this study experienced increased sexual interest after menopause.

Changes in sexual functioning are best assessed by longitudinal studies. A critical appraisal of the literature requires consideration of both biological and sociocultural influences on the researchers and the study subjects. McCoy et al. (1985) documented a significant decline in rates of sexual intercourse in women followed up from 2 years' premenopause to 1.5 years' postmenopause. This decline was accompanied by a statistically significant decrease in circulating levels of both testosterone and estradiol.

Hawton et al. (1994) studied sexual function in a randomly selected community sample of 436 middle-aged women and their partners in the United Kingdom. Frequency of sexual intercourse and orgasm, enjoyment of sexual activity with a partner, and sexual satisfaction in the women were most clearly related to "marital adjustment." The woman's age and her partner's age were factors in frequency of sexual activity.

Hagstad and Janson (1984) and Hällström and Samuelsson (1990) reported on studies of Swedish women. Hagstad and Janson noted a gradual decline in ovarian estrogen secretion and stable androgen secretion in women older than 40. These women reported unchanged or increased sexual interest. This finding was attributed by the authors to sexual activity being important to the women's relationships. Hällström and Samuelsson evaluated 677 middle-aged women from the general population regarding their sexual desire on two occasions 6 years apart. Sexual desire showed considerable stability over time. Twenty-seven percent of the women reported a decrease in interest, and 10% had an increase in desire between the two interviews. Age, quality of the relationship, and mental health were major contributing factors toward change in desire in both directions.

Dennerstein et al. (1994) conducted a cross-sectional survey of 2,001 randomly selected Australian women between ages 45 and 55. The focus of this study was change in sexual interest over the previous 12-month period. More than 60% of the subjects reported no change in sexual interest. Thirty-one percent of the subjects reported a decrease in sexual desire associated with natural menopause, physical disorders, decreased employment, and physical symptomatology (vasomotor, cardiopulmonary, and skeletal).

Sarrel (1990) interviewed 185 women attending a menopause clinic in London, England. Of these women, 86.5% reported a sexual problem during sexual history taking. Of the problem group, 45% had desire phase disorders: 36% with excitement phase disorders and 27% with orgasmic phase disorders. Dyspareunia was reported by 43% of the women with problems (50% had secondary vaginismus). Twenty-three percent acknowledged a sexual dysfunction in their male partner.

In a previous study, Sarrel (1982) evaluated 50 couples, in which all women were postmenopausal, presenting for sexual counseling. He found that the problem was shared by men and women in 60%, was identified as female in 22%, and was identified as male in 18% of couples.

Masters (1986) reported a 60% response to therapy in anorgasmic postmenopausal women. He concluded that the best insurance for continued sexual ability in later years appears to be frequent sexual activity between ages 20 and 40. He stated that continued sexual activity in later years maintains normal function but also protects against the involutional changes caused by the decline in sex steroids.

In summary, this literature reports that a gradual decrease in sexual desire accompanies natural menopause in a proportion of women. It is not clear whether this decline relates to natural aging, biological changes at menopause, or the sociocultural context within which this transition occurs. Other women report unchanged or improved sexual lives during or after menopause. The male partner, if present, appears to play a key role in continuation or cessation of sexual activity in some relationships.

Sexual Dysfunction

Case 1

Ms. A, a 52-year-old postmenopausal woman, was referred for a second opinion because of complaints of painful intercourse and a dry vagina. Her last menstrual period was 3 years ago, and she has had increasing difficulties with intercourse since that time. She saw her gynecologist 6 months ago and was given a diagnosis of atrophic vaginitis. Hormone replacement therapy was initiated, and she noticed some early improvement in vaginal lubrication but has had persistent discomfort during intercourse. Sexual desire and response were satisfactory.

On pelvic examination, Ms. A was found to have vaginismus. This secondary vaginismus was induced by repeated painful attempts at intromission while she had vaginal atrophy caused by low estrogen levels. Simple Kegel and reverse Kegel exercises[1] while using her own lubricated fingers as a dilator were enough to reassure her of the potential for coital comfort, and the problem resolved.

Intrapersonal Factors

Many personal factors play an important role in a woman's adaptation to the transition through the climacteric. During this time, she may be adjusting to many other life changes (see Gise, Chapter 3, and Charney and Stewart, Chapter 8, in this volume). Other life stressors affecting women at this stage in their life may include health problems, children's leaving or returning home, responsibility for the care of parents, career difficulties, family conflicts, or financial problems (see Chapter 3). These stressors may affect their libido. Her ability to adjust will depend partly on whether she views menopause as another sign of aging or experiences it as a liberation. North American culture does not see aging as a positive life experience.

Case 2

Ms. B, a 56-year-old woman, was referred with a history of lack of sexual desire, which dated back to her menopause 4½ years ago. She had not taken any hormone replacement therapy and had not had any vasomotor symptoms of menopause. She had not had intercourse for 3 years and had no interest in self-pleasure. Her primary reason for attending is that she felt that continued lack of interest would pose a threat to her relationship unless she could recover some interest in sexual function. She described her partner as involved and caring, and he had made no threats or accusations.

During the first three interviews, Ms. B talked of her sadness resulting from a sense of emptiness in her life. Her children were both attending universities, her parents and other family members were in Scotland, and she felt that her body was falling apart. She admitted to sleep disturbance, profound sadness, lack of

---

[1] Kegel and reverse Kegel exercises are designed to establish voluntary control over the pelvic floor muscles. Kegel exercise involves contraction of the muscle, whereas reverse Kegel exercise is a quick contraction followed by a conscious 5- to 10-second relaxation of the muscle.

energy and interest in any daily activity, and weight gain of 20 pounds over the last 2 years. In retrospect, she believed that her problems began at menopause and that since then her usefulness as a woman had ended. With psychotherapy and antidepressant medication, her depression diminished and libido improved, and she became more sexually active.

Relationship Factors

Relationships can significantly affect a woman's ability to cope with the transition of the climacteric. Women who are divorced, widowed, and unemployed and who lack social support may have great difficulty in coping with these life stressors (see Chapter 3). Strong social supports, financial and employment security, and an involved, supportive partner have a significant and positive effect on a woman's ability to deal with the stresses of menopause (Carter 1995; Leysen 1995). Women who have a sense of competence, autonomy, and esteem and a positive attitude toward their sexuality throughout life are more likely to experience intimacy in their relationships with their mates than are women without these qualities. Consistent congruent communication and negotiation skills set the stage for intense and self-sustaining intimacy and sexual pleasure. If partners are uncommunicative, chauvinistic, and remote, the relationship is likely to deteriorate and sexual desire wane. In this situation, women often look to their children for emotional support. The empty nest at the time of menopause can produce a heightened sense of vulnerability for these women (Misri 1995).

Case 3

Ms. C, a 49-year-old woman, complains of perimenopausal bleeding. At the end of her recent visit, she expressed concern about her lack of sexual interest, difficulty with arousal, and inability to achieve orgasm during the last 3 years. She stated that her husband wonders whether these problems are the result of her menopause. On inquiry, she admitted to a chronically conflicted relationship, lack of problem resolution, unfulfilling sexual relationship, and a sense of isolation and emotional abuse.

Women who ask questions at the termination of their visit, or on behalf of a family member, require special attention and careful listening skills on the part of the clinician.

Ms. C's decline in sexual interest and arousability was a symptom of major relationship dysfunction. Biologically, she continued to have adequate levels of circulating sex steroids. Her husband was hoping to find an easy solution from the physician so he could continue to avoid facing the real problems in the relationship. After an individual assessment, the husband was invited for a conjoint assessment. They are currently in conjoint marital/sexual therapy.

Sexuality After Surgical Menopause

Surgical menopause creates a dramatic reduction in circulating estradiol, progesterone, and androgen levels. Prospective studies consistently report changes in sexual function subsequent to oophorectomy and hysterectomy. Despite the possible deleterious effects of oophorectomy on sexual desire and subjective arousal, physiological arousal, as measured by photoplethysmography, in women with surgical menopause did not differ from that in control subjects (Bellerose and Binik 1993). Women who have had hysterectomies may notice a dramatic change in their orgasmic response. This may be explained by the loss of uterine contractions, which have been an important part of their subjective experience of orgasm, as well as the possible role of "cervical tapping" in triggering coital orgasm (Cutler et al., in press). Subtotal hysterectomy has been reported to produce a less negative effect on sexual response than total hysterectomy (Kilkku 1983). Outcome seems to be related to the quality of sexual functioning before the operation, the patient's expectations of the effect of the operation on sexuality, and the lack of psychological preparation for the loss of the uterus. Hysterectomy and oophorectomy have the greatest effect on desire, orgasm, and coital comfort. Postoperative estrogen replacement enhances coital comfort but does not appear to enhance sexual function (Walling et al. 1990). Estrogen combined with androgen supplements improves a woman's energy and mood, as well as increases her sexual desire, sexual arousal, and frequency of fantasies (Sherwin and Gelfand 1987).

Treatment

The appropriate treatment of sexual problems during the transition to menopause requires a comprehensive assessment of the personal and relationship factors, hormonal status, and physical factors.

The assessment of personal factors may identify women who are facing the transition without supports or who are coping with personal crises in their lives and are, therefore, at increased risk for developing problems. If sexuality is a priority for them, *individual therapy* is indicated. The patient may benefit from a psychoeducational approach to psychotherapy that combines information about the biological aspects of menopause, the sociocultural context in which the transition occurs, and sexual socialization factors that may contribute to desire or arousal phase disorders at this time in her life. Lifestyle counseling includes protecting time for recreation and relaxation as well as time for erotic and sensuous pursuits. Helpful suggestions to promote sensuous reawakening can include aromatherapy, massage, music and dance, and self-pleasuring. Psychotherapeutic issues may include the meaning of sexuality, fertility, menopause, and aging to the woman and an exploration of issues in establishing a relationship with a partner, if that is of interest to her.

Conjoint sexual therapy may require a primary focus on rehabilitation of intimacy in the relationship. If the presenting complaint is a desire phase disorder in either of the partners, behavioral techniques as an initial approach are not helpful. This symptom requires the reestablishment of a degree of awareness of one's own sexuality and a desire to express that sexuality in the context of the relationship. Relaxation techniques, imaging, and renewal of courtship behaviors help to initiate the process. Once the couple shares the goal of mutual sexual pleasure, the first step is protecting time for intimacy. Sources of stress, fatigue, and preoccupation must be addressed. If anxiety is a significant component for one or both partners, systematic relaxation techniques will be helpful. Once a good level of relaxation is achieved, imaging of romantic or sensuous activities can help in the transition to the renewal of courtship behaviors. Reading together (e.g., *The Joy of Sex* [Comfort 1972]) and

planning the exercise can help to reduce anxiety. Once both partners are interested and feel a sense of safety about the relationship,
sensate focus exercises are suggested. This activity involves communication and touching exercises in which coitus is initially
avoided. Each partner takes responsibility for verbal communication about his or her desire and where he or she wishes to be
touched and for feedback about the quality of the experience. This
allows each partner to learn how to pleasure and be pleasured with
a focus on verbal and nonverbal communication. Once these goals
are achieved, genital caresses are included, and, eventually, with
mutual consent, coitus is introduced when appropriate. The emphasis of therapy is helping the patient create a smorgasbord of
sensuous and sexual techniques that emphasize pleasure, not performance, as the goal of sexual interaction.

Discussion

The current state of knowledge and research does not fully eluci-
date the association between sexuality and menopause. Biological
changes at menopause that can affect sexual function are obscured
by cultural and relationship factors. Much of the literature focuses
on coital frequency to define sexual desire and coital discomfort to
define a sexual problem. Undue emphasis on a woman's role as
procreant and equating reproduction, sexual function, and intercourse may result in a woman's seeking an escape at menopause
from a repetitive and monotonous coital relationship. Many sexual
activities of a woman at menopause that do not involve a partner
seem relatively unaffected by this transition. Management of sexual
complaints in the perimenopausal patient and her partner involves
elements of education, endocrine assessment, psychoeducational
counseling, and, when indicated, individual or conjoint psychotherapy (see Stotland, Chapter 9, and Robinson and Stirtzinger,
Chapter 10, in this volume). Most patients and their partners can
benefit from relevant sex information and counseling. Major relationship dysfunction and women with depression or dysphoric disorders may require mental health treatment (see Charney and
Stewart, Chapter 8, and Stotland, Chapter 9, in this volume) before
sexual desire or function will improve. Further research of this

natural life event will help to clarify the many unanswered questions that define the effect of menopause on sexuality.

References

Bachmann GA: Estrogen-androgen therapy for sexual and emotional well-being. The Female Patient 18:35–42, 1993

Bancroft J: A physiological approach, in Theories of Human Sexuality. Edited by Geer JH, O'Donohue W. New York, Plenum, 1987, pp 411–421

Beach FA: Sexual attractivity, proceptivity and receptivity in female mammals. Horm Behav 7:105–138, 1976

Bellerose SB, Binik YM: Body image and sexuality in oophorectomized women. Arch Sex Behav 22:435–459, 1993

Carter D: Psychiatric disorders and menopause. Journal of the Society of Obstetricians and Gynecologists of Canada 17 (suppl):5–9, 1995

Comfort A (ed): The Joy of Sex. New York, Crown Publishing, 1972

Cutler W, Friedmann E, Genovese-Stone E: Sexual response in healthy women. (in press)

Dennerstein L, Smith AMA, Morse CA, et al: Sexuality and the menopause. J Psychosom Obstet Gynecol 15:59–66, 1994

Greenblatt R, Mortara F, Torpin R: Sexual libido in the female. Am J Obstet Gynecol 44:658–663, 1942

Hagstad A, Janson PO: Sexuality among Swedish women around forty—an epidemiological survey. J Psychosom Obstet Gynecol 3:191–203, 1984

Hällström T, Samuelsson S: Changes in women's sexual desire in middle life: the longitudinal study of women in Gothenburg. Arch Sex Behav 190:259–268, 1990

Hawton K, Gath D, Day A: Sexual function in a community sample of middle-aged women with partners: effects of age, marital, socioeconomic, psychiatric, gynecological, and menopausal factors. Arch Sex Behav 23:375–395, 1994

Kaplan HS, Owett T: The female androgen deficiency syndrome. J Sex Marital Ther 19:3–24, 1993

Kilkku P: Supravaginal uterine amputation vs. hysterectomy: effects on libido and orgasm. Acta Obstet Gynecol Scand 62:141–145, 1983

Kligman EW: Office evaluation of sexual function and complaints. Clin Geriatr Med 7:18–37, 1991

Lamont JA: Promoting sexual wellbeing in the elderly. Geriatrics 10:25–30, 1994

Lamont JA, Leitch R: Effects of oral contraceptives on the libido of older women. Journal of the Society of Obstetricians and Gynecologists of Canada 17 (suppl):1–6, 1995

Leysen B: Coping with the climacteric hormones and/or emancipation, in Abstracts 11th International Congress of Psychosomatic Obstetrics and Gynecology. Edited by Bitzer J, Stauber M. Basel, Switzerland, Monduzzi Editore, 1995, pp 461–466

Masters WH: Sex and aging—expectations and reality. Hosp Pract (Off Ed) 21:175–198, 1986

Masters WH, Johnson VE (eds): The aging female: anatomy and physiology, in Human Sexual Response. Boston, MA, Little, Brown, 1966, pp 223–238

McCoy NL, Davidson JM: A longitudinal study of the effects of menopause on sexuality. Maturitas 7:203–210, 1985

McCoy N, Cutler W, Davidson JM: Relationships among sexual behavior, hot flashes, and hormone levels in perimenopausal women. Arch Sex Behav 14:385–394, 1985

Misri S: Looking at menopause in a socio-cultural context. Journal of the Society of Obstetricians and Gynecologists of Canada 17 (suppl):1–4, 1995

Pfeiffer E, Davis GC: Determinants of sexual behaviour in middle and old age. J Am Geriatr Soc 20:151–158, 1972

Psarakis S, Devlin MC, Beckerson L: Menopause: a contemporary perspective. The Canadian Journal of OB/GYN 2:81–86, 1990

Roughan PA, Kaiser FE, Morley JE: Sexuality and the older woman. Clin Geriatr Med 9:87–106, 1993

Sarrel PM: Sex problems after menopause: a study of fifty married couples treated in a sex counseling programme. Maturitas 4:231–237, 1982

Sarrel PM: Sexuality and menopause. Obstet Gynecol 75 (4, suppl):26S–30S, 1990

Semmens JP, Wagner G: Estrogen deprivation and vaginal function in postmenopausal women. JAMA 248:445–448, 1982

Sherwin BB: Menopause and sexuality. The Canadian Journal of OB/GYN 4:254–260, 1992

Sherwin BB, Gelfand MM: The role of androgen in the maintenance of sexual functioning in oophorectomized women. Psychosom Med 49:397–409, 1987

Walling M, Andersen BL, Johnson SR: Hormonal replacement therapy for postmenopausal women: a review of sexual outcomes and related gynecologic effects. Arch Sex Behav 19:119–137, 1990

Winn RL, Newton N: Sexuality in aging: a study of 106 cultures. Arch Sex Behav 11:283–298, 1982

CHAPTER 6

Medical Management: Individualizing Care for the Menopausal Patient

Harriette R. Mogul, M.D., M.P.H.

*T*he medical evaluation of menopausal women is receiving increased recognition for two reasons: 1) an awareness of the profound effects of hormonal decline on the major causes of mortality for older women and 2) the importance of assessing individual benefits and risks of estrogen for women contemplating postmenopausal hormone replacement therapy (HRT) in view of increasing evidence associating long-term estrogen use with an increased incidence of breast cancer in a small but statistically significant number of women.

Although concern about the relationship between estrogen replacement therapy (ERT) and breast cancer is not new, controversy surrounding the long-term use of HRT was catapulted into the national spotlight with the 1995 publication of a report from the Nurses Health Study in the *New England Journal of Medicine* (Colditz et al. 1995). This analysis of breast cancer incidence in more than 120,000 nurses reported an increased relative risk of breast cancer secondary to the use of ERT in three categories of patients: 1) women who used estrogen for more than 5 years, 2) women who initiated therapy at an older age, and 3) women who used progestins. Moreover, these effects were additive. The study generated an outcry among countless women who were currently taking estrogen; menopausal HRT became front-page news, culminating in a *Time* magazine cover story. As a result, women in their 40s through their 70s have begun to question the knee-jerk prescription for conjugated equine estrogens and medroxyprogesterone acetate (MPA) as estrogen levels decline and gonadotropins soar. Perimenopausal women who are considering ERT and women who have been using estrogen for a decade are turning to physicians for renewed guidance. They view the decision to use estrogen as an important choice. They request a great deal of information and seek a more comprehensive evaluation of their individual overall risks for disorders associated with aging and hormonal decline. The so-called estrogen dilemma must be confronted by all physicians, as perimenopausal women come to them for assessment, advice, and answers.

Clearly, the importance of the correct evaluation of menopausal women transcends the recent media blitz on ERT. Menopause is a critical health milestone for women, and the manner in which physicians conceptualize and care for menopausal patients can be expected to have dramatic implications on the long-range health of a growing population of aging women. As about 40 million women approach menopause by the year 2000, all physicians must acquire a better understanding of the physiological changes and the long-range health implications associated with this important "passage" for women. Physicians in all disciplines must become familiar with an increasing variety of therapeutic options—hormonal and nonhormonal—that have potential effects on the age-related morbidity and mortality from those medical conditions that compromise the health of older women.

In this chapter, I highlight findings from relevant research to expand the knowledge base of clinicians, and introduce an approach to the menopausal patient that can be used by all physicians. An algorithm (see Figure 6–1) is provided as a guide to improve decisions about the appropriateness, timing, and duration of hormonal therapies. An impressive body of research has emerged in the past decade. Knowledge of the epidemiology, diagnosis, and treatment of conditions such as coronary artery disease and osteoporosis, as well as the risks and benefits of various hormonal regimens, gleaned from such studies will allow us to target therapies correctly. Clinical decisions cannot be made in a vacuum, and physicians in all specialties can benefit from information derived from research data. The potential for an increased risk of breast cancer in women who take long-term estrogen must be balanced against two decades of research that indicate that estrogen use is associated with improved quality and quantity of life for many women. Decreased death from coronary artery disease, lowered risk of hip and spine fractures, and a decrease in what is known as "all-cause" mortality have been reported in well-designed, prospective studies. A review of the latest research should enable clinicians to function more effectively and allow for more individualized care for their perimenopausal patients.

Individualizing care requires

- An appreciation of the potential benefits and risks of HRT in general and familiarity with the differences between various regimens
- Knowledge of alternatives to HRT for conditions that figure prominently in the future health of the average menopausal-age woman
- An algorithm for arriving at an individual risk-benefit analysis to target HRT appropriately

Clinical Decision Making About the Role of Hormonal Therapies

Knowledge of the causes of mortality in North American women influences clinical decision making and is an important first step in determining appropriate care for the menopausal patient.

Although cardiovascular disease is the number one killer of women and accounts for five times the number of annual deaths as breast cancer, it is still overlooked as a disorder of women. Cardiovascular diseases, which include heart disease and stroke, account for nearly 53% of all deaths in women older than 50 years compared with 4% of deaths due to breast cancer (Bush 1992). Nonetheless, women are far less concerned with the consequences of heart disease than those of breast cancer. Fear of breast cancer is a critical determinant of estrogen use for postmenopausal women and one of the most common reasons that women discontinue HRT, according to several studies on compliance. Ironically, some studies suggest that estrogen use may actually reduce all-cause mortality in certain categories of women with breast cancer (Cobleigh et al. 1994). A large randomized clinical trial is in progress at the M.D. Anderson Cancer Center to assess the role of estrogen in patients with a history of breast cancer.

Benefits of Hormone Replacement Therapy

Overall benefits of ERT from observation studies are summarized in Table 6–1.

Diminished All-Cause Mortality

Diminished all-cause mortality was demonstrated in a 1983 landmark prospective study of women from the Lipid Research Clinics. Four categories of women who were using ERT were compared with women who did not use estrogen. The relative risk as an outcome measure indicated that of all women who were current estrogen users, women who had undergone a hysterectomy and oophorectomy had the lowest age-specific mortality, followed by women who had a hysterectomy, and then women who did not have a hysterectomy (Bush et al. 1983).

Table 6–1.   Benefits of estrogen replacement therapy

Diminished all-cause mortality
Diminished cardiovascular mortality
Decreased stroke prevalence
Reduced risk of osteoporosis, increased bone mass, decreased fracture risk
Genitourinary effects
Diminished vasomotor symptoms
Improved quality of life
Cognitive benefits

Decreased Cardiovascular Mortality and Stroke Prevalence

The association of estrogen deficiency and heart disease was further strengthened by a 1987 report of the Nurses Health Study, which reported an increased risk of cardiovascular disease in women with early menopause (Colditz et al. 1987). In 1991, a 10-year follow-up study of this cohort showed decreased cardiovascular mortality in women taking estrogen, with an overall relative risk of heart disease of .56 (Stampfer et al. 1991).

At present, 16 (of 17) prospective epidemiological studies reported between 1971 and 1991 demonstrated decreased cardiovascular mortality, using all relevant outcomes, such as fatal and nonfatal myocardial infarction. Results of these studies are summarized in several reviews (Barrett-Connor and Bush 1991; Kuhn and Rackley 1993; Stampfer and Colditz 1991) and indicate an overall 50% reduction in cardiovascular mortality with estrogen use. Although none of these studies are randomized clinical trials of HRT, in contrast to the Women's Health Initiative—the $625 million multicenter study begun in 1992—the data are highly consistent. These findings figure prominently in recommendations of the American College of Physicians (Grady et al. 1992) and two *New England Journal of Medicine* editorials (Belchetz 1994; Davidson 1995), which advocate ERT for women with risk factors for coronary artery disease.

Research on women undergoing coronary angiography studies further supports the protective role of estrogen. All studies reported a lower prevalence of occlusive disease in estrogen users compared with non–estrogen users. For example, 22% of women using estrogen compared with 68% of women not using estrogen had evidence of significant coronary artery disease as defined by coronary vessel (luminal) diameter (Hong et al. 1992). A multicenter, randomized clinical trial was initiated in 1993 to ascertain the role of estrogen in reversing angiographically demonstrable coronary artery disease.

Animal and human studies indicate a variety of possible mechanisms by which estrogen reduces adverse cardiovascular events. Data from these studies support the conclusions of earlier epidemiological and angiographic studies and strengthen the causal

relationship between estrogen use and diminished risk of cardiovascular disease. A review of the multiple sites of estrogen action
on lipoproteins, blood pressure, vascular endothelial factors, lipogenesis, and coagulation studies is beyond the scope of this chapter. At least nine independent sites of action of estrogen have been
demonstrated and reported in peer-reviewed journals. These effects are summarized and referenced in Table 6–2.

Initially, the cardioprotective effect of estrogen was postulated
to be mediated predominantly through the creation of a "beneficial" lipid profile in which high-density lipoprotein (HDL) cholesterol was increased and low-density lipoprotein (LDL) and total
cholesterol were decreased (Walsh et al. 1991). As noted in Table
6–2, more recent data support a multifactorial role of estrogen in
the reduction of cardiac risk. Accordingly, newer studies suggest
that estrogen has multiple and, presumably, synergistic effects on
the entire process of atherogenesis, in addition to independent effects that cause dilation of both coronary and peripheral vascula-

---

Table 6–2.   Cardioprotective effects of estrogen

Improved lipoprotein profile: decreased total cholesterol and
   low-density lipoprotein and increased high-density lipoprotein levels
   (Walsh et al. 1991)
Increased vasodilation of coronary arteries as demonstrated in
   • Flow studies in monkey models (Williams et al. 1992)
   • Human Doppler-derived parameters (Gilligan et al. 1994)
Improved clearance of postprandial intermediate-density lipoproteins
   and chylomicron remnants and diminished lipogenesis in the
   endothelial vessel wall (Sack et al. 1994)
Decreased angiographically demonstrable coronary vessel occlusion
Improved exercise stress testing based on treadmill studies of female
   patients: specifically, fewer ischemic electrocardiogram changes,
   longer duration on treadmill (Rosano et al. 1993)
Decreased fibrinogen levels
Increased vasodilation of peripheral blood vessels (Volterrani et al.
   1995)
Improved action on vascular prostaglandins (Stanczyk et al. 1995)
Decreased response to stress (Lindheim et al. 1992) and arithmetic
   stress testing (Del Rio et al. 1994)

---

ture. The latter effects, demonstrated in two experimental settings (i.e., as an acute response to estrogen administration and secondary to chronic estrogen therapy), add further credibility to the use of estrogen in reducing cardiovascular mortality and provide biological plausibility, which is a critical ingredient for the establishment of causality in epidemiological research (Rothman 1986).

In summary, a considerable body of evidence now suggests a potential role of estrogen in reducing the number one cause of mortality in women. This evidence includes several individual benefits attributable to estrogen through specific animal and human studies and a strong overall benefit of estrogen in reducing cardiovascular mortality in prospective epidemiological studies. Physicians caring for menopausal women must be aware of the benefits of estrogen for women with known heart disease and the importance of identifying predisposed women through a systematic appraisal of relevant cardiovascular risk factors.

Reduced Risk of Osteoporosis

Osteoporosis, a disorder of low bone mass and microarchitectural deterioration of bone tissue, is an important complication of estrogen deficiency. Age-related decreases in bone density accelerate with menopause in all women and result in hip and spine fractures, which have dramatic social and economic effects. Costs associated with the care of hip fractures in the United States approximate $13 billion annually. Such fractures are associated with a 1-year mortality of 25% in 80-year-old women and have important social implications: more than 25% of affected women must give up their independent status and enter nursing homes (Kanis et al. 1994). Few practicing physicians are aware of recent advances in the diagnosis and prevention of osteoporosis. Progress in understanding normal bone metabolism and delineating the specific mechanisms of risk factors, such as smoking, alcohol use, and estrogen deficiency, in the pathogenesis of osteoporosis has contributed greatly to the understanding of the pathophysiology of the disorder.

An assessment of a patient's specific risk for osteoporosis using new definitions, diagnostic modalities, and therapies is an important aspect of the overall evaluation of the menopausal patient. The risk of osteoporosis increases dramatically with menopause, and this condition remains a major indication for medical intervention in the form of preventive therapy. Despite advances in the knowledge of osteoporosis, significant gaps persist in the area of risk prediction. Although it is generally appreciated that thinness, sedentary lifestyle, smoking, alcohol use, a diet deficient in calcium and/or vitamin D, and the use of certain medications are associated with diminished bone density and increased fracture risk, the determination of a given person's composite risk based on presence of specific putative risk factors is not possible. In contrast, in patients with cardiovascular disease, information on the presence of individual risk factors such as high blood pressure and cholesterol can be incorporated into statistical models to provide a summary of the probability of specific coronary artery disease outcomes, such as myocardial infarction. The absence of sensitive predictive models of osteoporosis translates into an increased need to perform bone density studies on large numbers of menopausal women.

The importance of bone densitometry is further underscored by new definitions of osteoporosis that emerged after the 1991 World Health Organization consensus conference (Kanis et al. 1994). Accordingly, diagnostic criteria for levels of osteoporosis are based on bone mineral density (BMD) measurements obtained with dual X-ray absorptiometry (DXA) technology; the patient's bone mineral content is compared with the mean value of a standard reference population. In the new diagnostic categories, "mild" osteoporosis is defined as a BMD between 1 and 2.5 standard deviations (SDs) below young adult mean, and moderate to severe "osteoporosis" is equivalent to a BMD more than 2.5 SDs below young adult mean. These measurements allow physicians to determine the presence and exact degree of osteoporosis and the probability of fracture in patients of all ages but that are particularly relevant for the menopausal woman. New biochemical markers of bone turnover represent additional useful modalities for the diagnosis of osteoporosis and other metabolic bone disorders.

The role of bone densitometry and biochemical markers in assessing the risk of osteoporosis in peri- and postmenopausal women remains controversial. Because bone densitometry defines the disorder and determines the exact probability for fracture risk, it is advocated by a growing number of physicians as part of the evaluation of all women in the menopausal transition. The urinary n-telopeptide (NTX), a new, simple, inexpensive, and highly sensitive test for increased bone resorption, could be incorporated into this assessment in view of its high correlation (.7) with bone density. Preliminary studies on the NTX indicate that a value greater than 40 on the second voided urine specimen of the day is associated with abnormal bone resorption in the postmenopausal woman. Thus, a reasonable algorithm might include the use of DXA in all menopausal women with any combination of risk factors suggestive of osteoporosis and the use of NTX to screen women without apparent risk. By this two-stage diagnostic process, baseline bone density measurements are obtained in most menopausal women, but unnecessary studies are avoided. The high sensitivity of the NTX should identify those patients who are apparently at low risk for osteoporosis and who would have been missed yet avoids the cost of performing DXAs on every patient. A second NTX after a 3-month interval can be used to reevaluate women with an initial normal bone density measurement who might be in the category of "fast bone losers" (35% of all menopausal women); it can also be used to assess change and monitor treatment response.

Hormonal therapy decreases bone resorption by mechanisms that are now well understood (Manolagas and Jilka 1995). It is an important therapeutic measure for osteoporosis and is the current cornerstone of treatment (see Shapiro, Chapter 7, in this volume). Although other antiresorptive measures (e.g., calcitonin) and the first-generation bisphosphonates (e.g., etidronate) have been used in women who cannot tolerate hormonal therapy, estrogen has been the primary treatment. This is because of the magnitude of estrogen's effect, which until recently was not matched by other regimens, and its ease of use (e.g., calcitonin had to be given by injection, and etidronate could not be used continuously because of its potential for bone demineralization). Additional new therapies received approval by the U.S. Food and Drug Administration (FDA) in 1995. These therapies will begin to gain ground as therapeutic agents of choice for the treatment of osteoporosis in women, particularly in women who wish to avoid long-term ERT. These agents include 1) slow-release oral fluoride, 2) newer second-generation bisphosphonates (e.g., alendronate sodium), and 3) nasal calcitonin.

Fluoride, which had shown promise as a bone-formation agent, had not been widely used because of a high incidence of side effects, particularly gastrointestinal disturbances, and a lack of effect in decreasing bone fracture rates. Modifications in the oral delivery system, which diminished side effects and which improved efficacy in reducing fractures, provide important incentives to reconsider its use.

Second-generation bisphosphonates are considerably more effective (by a 500-fold difference) than first-generation agents (e.g., etidronate) in increasing bone density as a result of a greater antiresorptive action. Second-generation bisphosphonates can be used continuously because of a diminished potential for bone demineralization compared with etidronate. These medications may be preferable to estrogen for some patients: women with little apparent risk for cardiovascular disease and women who are concerned about long-term use of ERT because of fear of breast cancer. Newer therapies—including intermittent low-dose parathyroid hormone, estrogen analogues such as raloxifen, and growth agents such as human-recombinant growth hormone and insulin-like growth factor (IGF)-1—are under investigation in a variety of clinical trials. Although these therapies are still experimental, they can be expected to increase preventive and therapeutic options for future menopausal women at risk for osteoporosis and fractures.

Although calcium and vitamin D therapy does not have a primary role in increasing bone mass in women with postmenopausal osteoporosis, except in rare cases of significant deficiency states, their use is advocated to prevent bone resorption. A dietary assessment can be used to calculate an appropriate recommendation for calcium supplementation. Typical requirements are 1,500 mg/day of calcium plus 400–800 U of vitamin D. Calcium, in the form of calcium carbonate or citrate, should be given at bedtime to maximize the effect on calcium economy by diminishing urinary excretion. Determinations of vitamin D (25-OH vitamin D_3) may be obtained if vitamin D deficiency is suspected, although its deficiency is more problematic in older patients who may have age-related impairment in the conversion of vitamin D skin precursors. A level below 30 is abnormal and suggests that supplementation with 800 IU may be preferable. Measurement of the active form of vitamin D (1,25 di-OH vitamin D_3) is rarely indicated in the care of the typical menopausal patient. Its measurement should be limited to patients with suspected hyperparathyroidism (in which the level is elevated) or patients taking medications, such as dilantin, phenobarbital, and steroids, that are known to induce vitamin D abnormalities.

Exercise, proper diet, smoking cessation, and alcohol moderation can enhance skeletal integrity and are important adjuncts to medical management (see Chapter 7). Physicians can help to maintain the skeletal health of their patients by educating them about the availability of new diagnostic and therapeutic measures to identify and treat patients with osteoporosis. Patients should be encouraged to adopt lifestyle modifications that may improve their general well-being in addition to their skeletal health.

Additional Benefits of Estrogen Replacement

Recent studies suggest additional benefits of postmenopausal estrogen. These benefits include antianxiety effects (Del Rio et al. 1994) and metabolic effects. Because women who use estrogen may be intrinsically healthier and wealthier (at least as determined by socioeconomic status and other baseline characteristics) than women who do not use estrogen, such effects may reflect a selection bias rather than a true metabolic effect. Additional studies are needed to delineate possible beneficial metabolic effects of estrogen that have potential importance to the long-range health of older women.

Risks of Estrogen Replacement Therapy

ERT has been associated with an increased risk of a number of medical conditions (Table 6–3). The long-awaited results of the Postmenopausal Estrogen/Progestin Interventions (PEPI) Trial demonstrated unequivocally that unopposed estrogen is associated with endometrial carcinoma (The Writing Group for the PEPI Trial

Table 6–3.	Risks of estrogen use

Uterine cancer[a]
Breast cancer[b]
Hypertriglyceridemia (oral estrogen), pancreatitis
Hypertension (selected patients)

[a]The Writing Group for the PEPI Trial 1995.
[b]Colditz et al. 1995.

1995). Patients receiving unopposed estrogen had a 40% incidence of endometrial hyperplasia, a precursor to cancer of the endometrium. The implications of this study suggest that all patients who have an intact uterus must be treated with a progestin. Approved regimens for progesterone include low-dose (e.g., 2.5 mg of MPA) continuous therapy or cyclical therapy for 14 days/month with a higher-dose regimen (either 5 or 10 mg of MPA) to induce withdrawal bleeding. Most patients prefer the continuous therapy, but "breakthrough" bleeding, particularly in the first 6 months of therapy, is a common problem in younger women (as compared with women who initiate therapy several years after menopause), which complicates management and may require switching to cyclical therapy.

There is no simple solution to sorting out the role of long-term ERT in breast cancer risk; breast cancer is multifactorial, and the clinician must evaluate numerous potential risk variables, including genetic predisposition, environmental exposures, and dietary factors. Until definitive data are available, physicians should modify recommendations for long-term ERT and base therapy on an individualized profile of risks and benefits. (See Chapter 7 for more information about breast cancer and estrogen.)

Estrogen Replacement Therapy and Women Older Than 65

As the list of benefits of long-term use of ERT lengthens, the issue of initiating therapy in women who are many years postmenopause is receiving increasing attention. Studies of estrogen use in the elderly indicate that ERT can be used safely and is well tolerated in this population. In fact, progesterone (which, as noted in the previous section, is a necessary companion medication to prevent endometrial hyperplasia in women who have not undergone hysterectomy) is less problematic in this age range than in younger women. The atrophic endometrium characteristic of older women permits the use of low-dose continuous progesterone because the frequency of typical breakthrough bleeding is decreased in this age range compared with younger women; this precludes the need for cyclical progesterone and avoids monthly withdrawal bleeding, which are among the most common reasons for discontinuing therapy in younger women. Documented effects of ERT with potential benefits for older women include cardiovascular benefits, improved skeletal integrity and diminished fracture risk, and cognitive benefits. One study among the community elderly indicated that women who use estrogen have lower rates of Alzheimer's disease, lower scores on dementia rating scales, and better performance on tests of cognitive skills than do women who do not use estrogen (Henderson et al. 1994). Decreased incidence of urinary tract infection is another important benefit of ERT in older women. Urinary incontinence affects 40% of postmenopausal women and is one of "the three leading causes for nursing home care" (Notelitz 1990, p. 240). HRT is reported to diminish symptoms in almost 50% of patients. Urosepsis is a frequent and serious complication of nursing home patients, and routine use of estrogen creams has been advocated in this population to improve integrity of the urogenital epithelium and decrease colonization of bacteria in the urethral wall. Oral estrogen may be more socially acceptable to nursing home patients than the alternative of nursing home attendants administering local applications of estrogen cream.

As with women of all ages contemplating the use of estrogen, potential benefits must be compared with potential risks, and universal use is not advocated. As noted earlier in this chapter, the recent Nurses Health Study report (Colditz et al. 1995) indicated an increased risk of breast cancer associated with long-term use of ERT in women older than 65. Other risks of oral estrogen can be particularly problematic in the older female population who have limited functional reserve. These risks include interaction with medications metabolized through the cytochrome P450 enzyme system, gallstones and biliary tract disease, increased triglycerides and secondary pancreatitis, thromboembolic phenomena, hypertension, decreased seizure threshold, and hepatic tumors.

In summary, estrogen's ability to decrease all-cause mortality, cardiovascular disease mortality, hip fracture, and urinary tract infection and to improve cognition suggests that it might well be considered an important adjunct to care in older female patients. Although few therapeutic modalities have equal potential to improve quality of life and decrease the incidence of a wide spectrum of common adverse medical conditions, concerns with the effect of medication side effects in this population require additional care in initiating and following HRT.

Individualizing Care: An Algorithm

A suggested approach to menopausal women separates post-menopausal HRT into considerations of the potential benefits of short-term and long-term use. Patients with menopausal symptoms who have no contraindications to estrogen use, such as current breast cancer, liver disease, or active thromboembolic disorders, may well benefit from HRT for up to 5 years (see section, "Short-Term Hormone Replacement," below). Long-term use of HRT should involve an evaluation of the individual patient's risk for key causes of mortality in women (i.e., heart disease, stroke, and cancer) plus a determination of specific risk of osteoporosis. Clinical decision making for the management of menopause is summarized in Figure 6–1.

Long-Term Hormone Replacement

In this algorithm, an individual risk-benefit analysis is determined by a consideration of the patient's underlying risk for coronary artery disease, osteoporosis, and breast cancer. This assessment should include 1) a family history of heritable causes of coronary artery disease, including presence of "premature" heart disease in mother, father, or sibling; familial lipid disorder; and predisposition to diabetes, hypertension, and obesity; and 2) an analysis of the

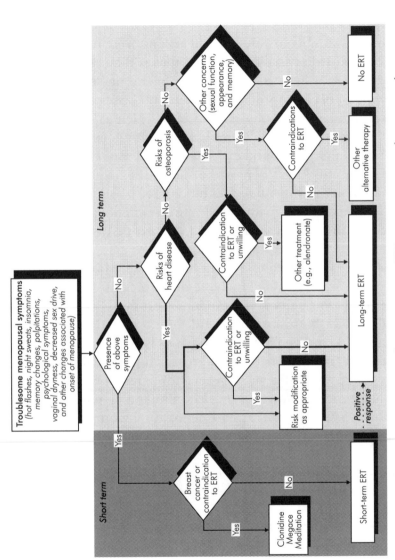

Figure 6–1. Decision tree for management of menopause. ERT = estrogen replacement therapy.

Source. Copyright © H. Mogul, M.D., M.P.H., P. Wynn, M.D., M.P.H.

patient's own cardiovascular risk profile obtained from baseline weight, body/mass index, fat disposition, blood pressure, lipid profile, blood sugar, and insulin action (if relevant) measurements. This assessment can provide a reasonable estimate of the risk of coronary artery disease outcomes.

The large number of independent actions of estrogen on factors that increase cardiovascular mortality makes the consideration of heart disease an important first step in the decision analysis. A growing list of cardioprotective benefits of estrogen accounts for increased advocacy by physician groups, such as the American College of Physicians, of HRT for women with documented heart disease or at high risk for heart disease. Physicians have a responsibility to identify these benefits to such patients and to provide information about the much greater danger posed by cardiovascular disease compared with breast cancer. Patients should be educated about the implications of such data so that they can make informed choices from available options.

A second consideration of long-term HRT involves the risk of osteoporosis as determined by bone densitometry and the use of specific biochemical markers for bone resorption. Patients should be advised that both hormonal and nonhormonal therapies are available for the prevention of menopausally related bone loss and the treatment of established osteoporosis. The availability of newer nonhormonal therapies such as second-generation bisphosphonates (alendronate), intranasal calcitonin, and slow-release fluoride provides options so that postmenopausal women can reduce their risk of fracture even if they have contraindications to hormones or concerns about the long-term safety of HRT.

The remaining category of indications for long-term HRT is listed as "other considerations." These include maintenance of youthful skin tone, libido, and sexual function; possible cognitive and affective benefits; and overall effects on well-being. The use of hormones to attenuate the inevitable consequences of aging is controversial for a variety of reasons. Clearly, such conditions are not life-limiting, and physicians and patients alike must decide whether long-term estrogen is warranted to address such symptoms. Second, there is an absence of consensus regarding therapeutic efficacy because of the paucity of studies to address the risk-benefit profile of long-term HRT for these indications. In the absence of specific contraindications to estrogen use, amelioration of age-related changes might serve as a basis for long-term HRT.

Short-Term Hormone Replacement

Short-term HRT for symptoms of menopause should be considered separately. This treatment option may be recommended with greater impunity because 1) ERT is not associated with an increased risk of breast cancer in the first 5 years of use (Colditz et al. 1995), and 2) HRT is currently the most effective treatment for symptoms associated with the onset of menopause, such as hot flashes, night sweats, sleep deprivation associated with nighttime awakening, palpitations, and vaginal dryness. Alternative treatments have limited efficacy; for example, clonidine, a central α-adrenergic blocker, is effective in only 40% of patients. Other therapies such as megace (a progesterone derivative) and meditation, which have been reported in peer-reviewed journals; and vitamin therapies and other health remedies, which continue to receive recognition, have not been subjected to rigorous scientific study. Thus, care providers may wish to suggest the use of short-term HRT for treatment of symptoms associated with menopause, particularly when symptoms interfere with functioning and/or diminish quality of life.

Nonhormonal Approaches

Physicians from a wide variety of specialties should anticipate questions from peri- and postmenopausal women about the risks and benefits of hormonal and nonhormonal therapies for disorders associated with menopause and estrogen deficiency. These encounters provide an opportunity for clinicians to discuss not only HRT but also other lifestyle modifications appropriate for menopausal women. Patients at minimal risk for heart disease, particularly those with a strong family history of breast cancer and/or a constellation of risk factors associated with breast cancer (e.g., early menarche, obesity, nulliparity), or patients disinclined to take estrogen should be encouraged to consider nonhormonal therapies. All women with evidence of or risk factors for either heart disease or osteoporosis should be advised that irrespective of whether hormones are selected, lifestyle modification and/or preventive medical treatment of related risks may confer additional benefits. Accordingly, exercise, proper diet, and modification of smoking and alcohol intake should be advocated to reduce the risk of cardiovascular disease, although specific data on risk modification in women are not currently available. Medical management of hypertension and hyperlipidemia and programs for weight and smoking reduction can further enhance care for patients with relevant cardiovascular risk factors.

The following two cases involving two patients, Ms. A and Ms. B, provide contrasting examples of menopausal management:

Case 1

Ms. A, a 52-year-old lawyer and holocaust survivor, consulted a menopause health program because of severe hot flashes, insomnia, and palpitations. Review of symptoms indicated that she had moderate hypertension, which was poorly controlled, and panic attacks. Her panic attacks had been lifelong, since her adolescence in a concentration camp, but were not diagnosed until her late 30s after she read a description of the condition in the *New York Times,* which prompted her to seek consultation with a psychiatrist. After several years of psychotherapy and medication, the panic attacks had almost entirely abated; she took alprazolam only on an as-needed basis a few times a year.

Her menstrual periods were somewhat irregular, generally occurring every 30–45 days; menopausal symptoms included frequent hot flashes, night sweats, insomnia, and fatigue. She also noted palpitations, some memory loss, and a return of panic symptoms, which were now occurring on a regular basis about once per week, for which she had resumed medication with alprazolam.

Ms. A was interested in a menopause evaluation because she was troubled by symptoms of menopause and wondered about the possible relationship with the return of her panic attacks; she had also heard about the cardioprotective effects of estrogen. On physical examination, Ms. A was an attractive, but slightly unkempt, woman who was pleasant but somewhat ill at ease and visibly nervous. Her blood pressure was 140/92 mm Hg and pulse was 80 with occasional extrasystole. Examination of her heart revealed a soft systolic murmur, and breast examination indicated a few small cysts bilaterally in the upper outer quadrants. The remainder of the examination was entirely within normal limits. Laboratory findings included total cholesterol 246 mg/mL, LDL 170 mg/mL, normal serum chemistries, follicle-stimulating hormone (FSH) 85.5 ng/dL, luteinizing hormone (LH) 73 ng/dL, and estradiol 22 ng/dL; bone density indicated a T-score of −2.2 at the lumbosacral spine (total) and −1.83 at the hip. Electrocardiogram showed early left ventricular hypertrophy without ischemic changes. Pap smear and mammogram were within normal limits.

Ms. A was anxious to see whether estrogen could ameliorate her hot flashes and insomnia. Her elevated cholesterol level and bone density findings (mild osteoporosis almost meeting criteria for moderate osteoporosis at the spine) provided additional reasons to consider estrogen. The physician prescribed an estrogen patch 0.05 mg/day, calcium citrate 1,000 mg/day, and vitamin D 800 U and advised her to return in 1 month for evaluation of blood pressure and initiation of progesterone (which was deferred for 1 month to evaluate her blood pressure and mood response to unopposed estrogen).

The most striking aspect of Ms. A's return visit was the transformation in her appearance, which was noted by the entire office staff. She had lightened and permed her hair, was wearing makeup and new clothing, and was considerably less nervous than during her previous visit. She stated that she felt "absolutely wonderful," with her new-found energy level and general sense of well-being. She reported some skin irritation with the patch and was advised to change the location to her buttocks, because fewer skin reactions occur at this site. Her blood pressure was 130/85, and repeat total cholesterol was 223, with an LDL cholesterol of 146. She was given a 3-month prescription for MPA 2.5 mg/day and advised to return to her primary care physician for additional management of her hypertension and hyperlipidemia.

Six weeks later, Ms. A called to report a severe reaction to the patch: a 4-cm localized swelling, which was hot, tender, and erythematous; generalized swelling of the surrounding buttocks and upper leg; and fever of 101°F, with generalized malaise. She had discontinued the patch and was experiencing severe hot flashes. The physician prescribed conjugated equine estrogen to be taken when she was feeling completely well in half the dose

(0.3 mg) and then, if tolerated, as a full dose. She was instructed to discontinue therapy if any adverse effects occurred. She initially did very well on oral medication, with full return to her former estrogen-replete state. Some weeks later, Ms. A called to report that she had experienced two episodes of acute-onset visual changes consisting of decreased vision with dancing spots associated with a mild headache and nausea. These episodes were not associated with a change in blood pressure, and she wondered whether they might be related to the estrogen. A neurological consultation confirmed the presence of "atypical migrainous optic syndrome" thought to be secondary to estrogen, and the symptoms abated with discontinuation of HRT.

Ms. A reconsulted the menopause program 6 months later because her hot flashes and insomnia had become increasing troublesome. At that time, various options, including clonidine, megace, and a new patch, were discussed. She was given a "skin test," which meant wearing the new patch on her hand for 4 and then 8 hours. No localized reaction was observed on her return visit, so the new patch was prescribed. At this writing, 1 year after the initiation of therapy, she feels well with no adverse skin or neuro-ophthalmological reactions.

Case 2

Ms. B, a 53-year-old secretary who had been taking estrogen for 6 months, sought consultation because she wondered whether "she really needed it." She had experienced no symptoms associated with menopause before starting HRT with oral estrogen plus cyclical progesterone (MPA 10 mg/day for 10 days/cycle). Family history indicated that her father had heart disease, with two myocardial infarctions before age 60. Ms. B's medical history was entirely unremarkable except for a long history of being significantly overweight, until age 38. At about that age, she began to work out at the fitness center on a daily basis and subsequently lost 25 pounds over the course of a year. Ms. B reported that she drank a quart of skim milk every day, took a multivitamin and antioxidant vitamins, and walked, hiked, or biked every day in addition to her hourly weight-training sessions. On physical examination, she was a well-muscled woman who looked many years younger than her stated age. She weighed 139 pounds and was 5 feet 7 inches tall. Her blood pressure was 115/75 mm Hg and pulse was

72 and regular. Physical examination was unremarkable except for bilateral cystic breasts. Laboratory findings included normal serum chemistries, including calcium 9.8, total cholesterol 173 mg/mL, HDL 91 mg/mL, and LDL 64 mg/mL; bone density indicated a T-score of −1.13 at the spine and −.29 at the hip.

We decided that Ms. B had no short- or long-term indications for HRT. She discontinued estrogen and progesterone and reported feeling even better because of decreased mood swings, which she had attributed to the progesterone. She stated that she lost 5 pounds without any dietary modification. Ms. B was advised to continue her current calcium intake without additional supplementation and to have a repeat bone density measurement or a urinary NTX in 1 year.

Medical Evaluation of Menopause

A systematic medical assessment of menopausal women provides a foundation to consider appropriate preventive strategies for menopausal symptoms. This evaluation, which is summarized in Table 6–4, involves a thorough history, including a detailed family

Table 6–4. Laboratory tests for evaluation of the menopausal woman

Chemistry profile (including calcium, phosphorus, liver function tests)

Fasting lipid profile (total cholesterol, low-density lipoprotein cholesterol, high-density lipoprotein cholesterol, triglyceride levels)

Follicle-stimulating hormone, luteinizing hormone, estradiol (if perimenopausal or uncertain about menopause stage) measurements

Bone density (dual X-ray absorptiometry [DXA] is the "gold standard")

Urinary n-telopeptide (NTX) to establish baseline bone turnover and rule out "fast bone losers"

25-OH vitamin D (1,25 di-OH vitamin D_2, parathyroid hormone if hyperparathyroidism suspected)

Thyroid function tests (total and free thyroxine, thyroid-stimulating hormone) or urine pregnancy test (to eliminate nonmenopausal etiology for oligomenorrhea) if clinically appropriate

Fasting and 2-hour postprandial blood glucose and insulin level (if clinically indicated)

history that focuses on the risks for conditions associated with estrogen deficiency (e.g., osteoporosis and heart disease). Questions about the specific risks for these conditions in affected relatives are very important, because the presence of a disorder may relate to either heritable or nonheritable causes. For example, the implications of heavy tobacco use, obesity, and sedentary lifestyle in a family member with an early heart attack are clearly important and modify our interpretation of the apparent genetic risk for premature heart disease. A dietary history noting the number of dairy servings per day is useful to establish an approximate daily calcium intake.

Patients need a complete physical examination to determine general health status and focus on potential conditions that might modify recommendations for hormonal or nonhormonal therapies. For example, leg veins and the right upper quadrant of the abdomen should be examined to rule out active deep vein phlebitis and hepatobiliary disease in patients for whom estrogen is being considered, and epigastric tenderness, a possible contraindication to alendronate treatment of osteoporosis, should be evaluated. Laboratory tests should encompass a general chemistry profile, including calcium and phosphorus levels; fasting lipid profile for total cholesterol, HDL and LDL cholesterol, and triglyceride levels; and if menopausal status is unclear FSH, LH, and estradiol levels. Bone densitometry using a DXA (the gold standard) and a urinary NTX are important determinants of the risk of osteoporosis. A 25-OH vitamin D level should also be obtained. Thyroid function tests and a pregnancy test are occasionally indicated to ascertain whether the patient's symptoms are nonmenopausal in origin. Fasting and 2-hour blood glucose with insulin levels are useful if the patient has any risk factors or clinical symptoms suggestive of type II diabetes, because this disorder may present at menopause.

Summary

In summary, physicians must broaden their conception of menopause to encompass the full range of medical and nonmedical interventions that can improve the latter one-third of life for postmenopausal women. Although an increasing body of research suggests that HRT may favorably affect specific medical conditions, such as coronary artery disease and osteoporosis, that can diminish the quality and quantity of life for older women, other therapeutic options should also be promoted. Universal regimens that either advocate or preclude HRT for all menopausal women have no place in the physician's approach to the menopausal patient. Until long-term studies have fully elucidated the putative role of HRT in breast cancer, physicians should limit HRT to women who have clearly defined benefits based on a comprehensive analysis of specific individual risk for those disorders that compromise morbidity and mortality in aging women. All patients, especially women with contraindications to hormonal treatment, should be encouraged to adopt additional health-enhancing strategies, which may diminish the incidence of cardiovascular disease and hip fractures. Physicians are in a unique position to enlighten menopausal patients and provide a forum for discussion about critical physical health and mental health issues. Collectively, physicians can affect the quality and quantity of the postmenopausal years for countless women.

References

Barrett-Connor E, Bush TL: Estrogen and coronary heart disease in women. JAMA 265:1861–1867, 1991

Belchetz PE: Hormonal treatment of postmenopausal women. N Engl J Med 330:1062–1071, 1994

Bush T: The epidemiology of cardiovascular disease in postmenopausal women. Ann N Y Acad Sci 594:263–271, 1992

Bush TL, Cowan LD, Barrett-Connor E, et al: Estrogen use and all-cause mortality: preliminary results from the Lipids Research Clinics Program follow-up study. JAMA 249:903–906, 1983

Cobleigh MA, Berris RF, Bush TL: Estrogen replacement therapy in breast cancer survivors: a time for change. JAMA 272:540–545, 1994

Colditz GA, Willett WC, Stampfer MJ, et al: Menopause and the risk of coronary heart disease in women. N Engl J Med 316:1105–1110, 1987

Colditz GA, Hankinson SE, Hunter DJ, et al: The use of estrogens and progestins and the risk of breast cancer in postmenopausal women. N Engl J Med 332:1589–1593, 1995

Davidson NE: Hormone replacement therapy—breast vs. heart vs. bone. N Engl J Med 332:1638–1639, 1995

Del Rio G, Velardo A, Zizzo G, et al: Effect of estradiol on the sympathoadrenal responses to mental stress in normal men. J Clin Endocrinol Metab 79:836–840, 1994

Gilligan DM, Quyyumi A, O'Cannon R, et al: Effects of physiological levels of estrogen on coronary vasomotor function in postmenopausal women. Circulation 89:2545–2551, 1994

Grady D, Rubin SM, Petitti DB, et al: Hormone therapy to prevent disease and prolong life in postmenopausal women. Ann Intern Med 117:1016–1037, 1992

Henderson VW, Paganini-Hill A, Emanuel CK, et al: Estrogen replacement therapy in older women: comparisons between Alzheimer's disease cases and non-demented control subjects. Arch Neurol 51:896–900, 1994

Hong MK, Romm PA, Reagan K, et al: Effects of estrogen replacement therapy on serum lipid values and angiographically defined coronary artery disease in postmenopausal women. Am J Cardiol 69:176–178, 1992

Kanis JA, Melton LJ, Christiansen C, et al: The diagnosis of osteoporosis. J Bone Miner Res 9:1137–1141, 1994

Kuhn FE, Rackley CE: Review article: coronary artery disease in women: risk factors, evaluation, treatment, and prevention. Arch Intern Med 153:2626–2636, 1993

Lindheim SR, Legro RS, Bernstein L, et al: Behavioral stress responses in premenopausal and postmenopausal women and the effects of estrogen. Am J Obstet Gynecol 167:1831–1836, 1992

Manolagas SC, Jilka RL: Mechanisms of disease: bone marrow, cytokines, and bone remodeling—emerging insights into the pathophysiology of osteoporosis. N Engl J Med 332:305–311, 1995

Notelitz M: Is there a need for menopause clinics? Ann N Y Acad Sci 592:239–241, 1990

Rosano GM, Sarrel PM, Poole-Wilson PA, et al: Beneficial effect of oestrogen on exercise-induced myocardial ischaemia in women with coronary artery disease. Lancet 342:133–136, 1993

Rothman KJ: Casual inference in epidemiology, in Modern Epidemiology. Boston, MA, Little, Brown, 1986, pp 16–20

Sack MN, Rader DJ, O'Cannon R: Oestrogen and inhibition of oxidation of low-density lipoproteins in postmenopausal women. Lancet 343:269–270, 1994

Stampfer MJ, Colditz GA: Estrogen replacement therapy and coronary heart disease: a quantitative assessment of the epidemiologic evidence. Prev Med 20:47–63, 1991

Stampfer MJ, Colditz GA, Willet WC, et al: Postmenopausal estrogen therapy and cardiovascular disease: ten-year follow-up from the Nurses Health Study. N Engl J Med 325:756–762, 1991

Stanczyk FZ, Rosen GF, Ditkoff EC, et al: Influence of estrogen on prostacyclin and thromboxane balance in postmenopausal women. Journal of the North American Menopause Society 2:137–143, 1995

Volterrani N, Rosano G, Coats A, et al: Estrogen acutely increases peripheral blood flow in postmenopausal women. Am J Med 99:119–122, 1995

Walsh BW, Schiff I, Rosner B, et al: Effects of postmenopausal estrogen replacement on the concentrations and metabolism of lipoproteins and apolipoproteins in postmenopausal dyslipidemic women. N Engl J Med 325:1196–1199, 1991

Williams JK, Adams MR, Herrinton DM, et al: Short-term administration of estrogen and vascular responses of atherosclerotic coronary arteries. J Am Coll Cardiol 20:452–457, 1992

The Writing Group for the PEPI Trial: Effect of estrogen or estrogen/progestin regimens on heart disease risk factors in postmenopausal women: the Postmenopausal Estrogen/Progestin Interventions (PEPI) Trial. JAMA 273:199–208, 1995

CHAPTER 7

Hormone Replacement Therapy

Heather M. Shapiro, M.D., F.R.C.S.C.

*I*n this chapter, I focus primarily on the practical consideration of hormone replacement therapy (HRT) (and some nonhormonal therapies for menopausal symptoms): how to determine the need, how to determine the best regimen, how to deal with effects, and when to start and stop HRT. The physiology, symptoms (see Baram, Chapter 2, in this volume), and medical evaluation and management of menopause (see Mogul, Chapter 6, in this volume) have been addressed in earlier chapters of this book. In this chapter, I briefly review these subjects as they apply to the decision-making process and concentrate on the effects of HRT. Like all medical decision making, the decision of whether to use HRT depends on the favorable balance between risk and benefit. Unlike some medical therapies, the outcome with HRT is multidimensional and fraught with a multitude of uncertainties.

HRT is used to describe various types and combinations of drugs, all of which have in common the presence of both an estrogen and a progestin. Estrogen replacement therapy (ERT), prescribed mostly for women who have had hysterectomies, contains estrogen only. An estimated 13.6 million prescriptions were dispensed for oral menopausal estrogens in 1982 in the United States. More than 31 million prescriptions were dispensed in 1992 (Wysowski et al. 1995). One in six to one in four postmenopausal women were taking menopausal hormones in 1992 in the United States. However, these seemingly low numbers may be misleading because in women aged 50–54 the rates approach 50%. Although it appears that HRT use is not widespread, these numbers suggest that use is increasing dramatically. Thus, it is imperative for all clinicians treating menopausal women to be aware of issues surrounding HRT. The common hormone preparations available are described in Table 7–1.

Recent attention has also been directed to the role of androgens in menopausal women. Traditionally, testosterone has been regarded as the male hormone and estrogen as the female hormone. However, androgens are also involved in female sexual behavior, affect, and cognitive function and contribute to the maintenance of muscle mass, pubic hair, and libido (Sands and Studd 1995; Sherwin et al. 1985).

Table 7–1.   Hormone preparations available

Product	Dose	Active substance	Side effects
CES, Premarin	0.3, 0.625, 0.9, 1.25, 2.5 mg	Conjugated estrogen	Breast tenderness, nausea, vaginal bleeding
Ogen	0.625, 1.5 mg	Estropipate	Breast tenderness, vaginal bleeding
Estinyl	20 µg/day	Ethinyl estradiol	Breast tenderness, vaginal bleeding
Estrace	1, 2 mg oral	17 β estradiol	Breast tenderness, vaginal bleeding
Estraderm	25, 50, 100 µg/day	17 β estradiol	Breast tenderness, vaginal bleeding, skin irritation
Provera	2.5, 5.0, 10.0 mg	Medroxy-progesterone acetate	Bloating, irritability, weight gain, headache
Micronor	0.15 mg	Norethindrone	Bloating, irritability, weight gain, headache
Prometrium	200, 300 mg	Oral micronized progesterone	Bloating, irritability, weight gain, headache

Note.   CES = congugated equine estrogen.

HRT is given most commonly in one of three regimens, as listed in Table 7–2. Any oral or transdermal estrogen or progestin can be used in any of the regimens.

Determining Need for Hormone Replacement Therapy

Medical Perspective: Practice Guidelines

Many physicians are theoretically in favor of HRT, but there is little consensus in determining which individuals require it (Campbell-Brown and McEwan 1992). One approach is to develop practice guidelines. Most professional associations have developed practice guidelines, including the American Society for Reproductive Medicine jointly with the American College of Cardiology. All are supportive of HRT, but the degree of support varies. Even when physicians' knowledge of outcome and probabilities matches that in the literature, the clinical decision is often different (Elstein et al. 1986). The biggest fear, for clinicians and patients alike, is cancer (Grady et al. 1992).

Societal Perspective: Cost-Effectiveness

Studies have estimated that various strategies for HRT could cost between $11,700 and $22,100 per year of additional life gained (Tosteson et al. 1990). If the cost of screening for osteoporosis is low,

Table 7–2.   Hormone replacement therapy regimens

Regimen	Schedule of estrogen	Schedule of progestin	Comment
Estrogen only	Daily	None	For women with hysterectomies
Cyclic	Daily	Days 1–12[a]	Preferred regimen
Cyclic	Days 1–25[a]	Days 15–25[a]	Traditional regimen
Continuous combined	Daily	Daily	Newer, fewer data

[a]Days of calendar month.

then resource savings from hip fractures prevented would be more than the cost of screening and treatment. Universal HRT without screening would prevent the most fatal fractures but would expose many more women to the adverse effects of HRT, with the attendant life-threatening risk of breast cancer. HRT is associated with increased quality of life, a large percentage of which is attributed to a relief of menopausal symptoms (Cheung and Wren 1992).

Individual Perspective

It is generally thought that a woman's decision to use HRT is based primarily on the need to relieve menopausal symptoms (Hammond 1994). Socioeconomic factors are also significant (Abraham et al. 1995; Thompson 1995). Some women might seek HRT at menopause to help alleviate preexisting emotional difficulties. For women without typical menopausal complaints, physicians prescribe HRT five times more often to those with a lower level of well-being. In some studies, women who intended to use HRT reported significantly lower self-esteem and higher levels of depressed mood, anxiety, and negative attitudes to the menopause. They also expressed stronger beliefs in their physician's ability, as opposed to their own, to control their menopause experience (Hunter and Liao 1994). However, the more common clinical perception is that women who approach their physician are making informed choices about HRT and, in fact, are improving their control as opposed to relinquishing it. Most still choose HRT for its short-term rather than long-term benefits (Roberts 1995). Women who choose not to use HRT usually do so because of a disinclination to use drugs and to interfere with a normal process, as well as concerns about vaginal bleeding and side effects (Cano 1994).

Treatment of Menopausal Symptoms

Hot flashes, sleep disorders, mood changes, menstrual changes, and genitourinary atrophy are the most common complaints of women in the climacteric (see also Baram, Lamont, Mogul, and Stotland, in Chapters 2, 5, 6, and 9, respectively, in this volume). Menopausal symptoms persist for longer than 1 year in more than 80%

of menopausal women and abate within 5 years in most women. The variability in symptoms among women is not clearly understood (Swartzman et al. 1990). To a certain degree, it is related to the absolute change in estradiol levels. Those women in whom the postmenopausal levels of estradiol are relatively higher than in other postmenopausal women will experience fewer hot flashes. In these women, the peripheral conversion of estradiol to estrogen is greater because of the larger amount of body fat, which is the site of the peripheral conversion. A variability in the hypothalamic sensitivity to the fluctuation of estradiol levels and in the inherent stability or instability of the thermoregulatory center is also likely. Hot flashes may be accompanied by sweating, chills, or anxiety. The variability in perception and distress associated with these changes certainly reflects individual and societal perspectives on menopause, but the relative contribution of each is unknown. The effect of symptoms on quality of life can be expressed as "quality-adjusted life years," and menopausal symptoms may be similar to a 20%–80% decrease in quality of life without hot flashes for some women (Daly et al. 1993).

Hot Flashes

Efficacy of Treatment

Hot flashes that are caused by low estrogen levels should theoretically be abated by the use of HRT (see also Chapters 2 and 6). Failure of therapy, ranging from 20% to 50%, may be a result of insufficient dose of estrogen (Steingold et al. 1985). This can be easily rectified by increasing the dose. Women receiving placebo treatment also improve, but their improvement is often short-lived.

Dose

The dose of estrogen required to abate hot flashes varies. The starting dose is usually the equivalent of 0.625 mg of conjugated equine estrogens. Higher doses are required when the endogenous circulating estradiol levels are low or when there has been an abrupt change in the levels. The first scenario is more common in thin women, particularly smokers, whereas the second is common in premenopausal women who have undergone surgical hysterectomy. There is no need to measure serum estradiol levels initially because the presence of hot flashes is a true bioassay for estrogen. There may be a role for measuring estradiol levels in women taking natural estrogen (e.g., not ethinyl estradiol or conjugated equine estrogens), in whom an increase in estradiol would be expected but hot flashes persist. If the levels are in the premenopausal range consistently, it may point to a nonmenopausal-related cause for the flashes.

Note that at no dose are the menopausal symptoms reduced 100%. This again confirms the multifactorial etiology of menopausal symptoms.

Regimen

All systemic HRTs are effective in alleviating hot flashes and other symptoms of hypoestrogenemia (Place et al. 1985). The choices should be based on side effects in the short term and consideration of long-term benefits of the different regimens. All available evidence suggests that, at equivalent doses, all estrogen preparations have equivalent effectiveness. Transdermal estrogen, although effective at alleviating hot flashes, is associated with up to a 20% incidence of skin reaction to the patch. Local therapy, by definition, only benefits symptoms of atrophic vaginitis. All other observed differences between the regimens appear to be idiosyncratic at this time.

Duration

When HRT is used for the treatment of hot flashes, it should be continued for 2 years, because this is the average duration of symptoms. If the symptoms recur and are disturbing when treatment is stopped, HRT should be reinstituted.

Nonhormonal Treatment

No nonhormonal treatments for hot flashes are as effective as estrogen (Limouzin-Lamothe et al. 1994). Clonidine (an α_2-adrenergic agonist) has been suggested as a treatment for hot flashes because of the presumed noradrenergic effect. It is also not contraindicated in patients with hormone-sensitive tumors. Several trials of clonidine for the treatment of hot flashes have shown a small and variable benefit. In a study of women with breast cancer (a contraindication to HRT) who were being treated with tamoxifen, clonidine did reduce frequency of hot flashes to a degree that was statistically significant ($P < .0001$) but clinically moderate (20% reduction from baseline). It also decreased severity of hot flashes by 10% from baseline. The authors concluded that a treatment better than clonidine is needed for patients in whom estrogen therapy is contraindicated (Goldberg et al. 1994).

Treatment of hot flashes with nonestrogens is significantly less effective than with estrogen. Danazol has been advocated as a treatment; however, only about 50% of women respond, and even then the hot flashes are not completely obliterated (Foster et al. 1985). Various dietary and herbal remedies have been advocated, but none has been the subject of controlled trials (see Jensvold, Chapter 11, in this volume). Environmental modifications (cooler clothing, dressing in layers, lower room temperature, fans, and avoiding caffeine and hot or spicy foods) may provide symptom relief for some women with mild or moderate symptoms.

Mood and Memory Changes

Efficacy of Treatment

The effects of menopause on mood and memory are often the most upsetting symptoms to women. The relationship between affective disorders and hypoestrogenemia, independent of other menopausal factors, is unclear. (The etiology of these changes and treatment options are discussed in Mogul, Charney and Stewart, and Stotland, Chapters 6, 8, and 9, respectively, in this volume.) Estrogen is purported to improve cognitive function. Verbal and spatial memory, language, attention, and general spatial skills may differ between HRT users and nonusers (Barrett-Connor and Kritz-Silverstein 1993; Kampen and Sherwin 1994). In patients with Alzheimer's disease, the effect of estrogen appears to be favorable, although the number of patients and the number of studies are small (Brenner et al. 1994; Henderson et al. 1994; Paganini-Hill and Henderson 1994).

Problems of Treatment

Virtually no studies address potential adverse cognitive or affective effects of HRT. Anecdotal evidence suggests that some women become depressed with the use of estrogen and progesterone, but this is not well documented in studies (Palinkas and Barrett-Connor 1992).

Special Considerations: Premenstrual Syndrome

Many clinicians are reluctant to prescribe HRT to women who have experienced premenstrual syndrome (PMS) premenopausally. However, women with a history of PMS had no significant difference in mood and physical symptoms when given HRT postmenopausally (Kirkham et al. 1991).

Further reassuring evidence of the safety of HRT in women with a history of PMS was shown by Mezrow et al. (1994) in a placebo-controlled trial. A gonadotropin-releasing hormone analogue (GnRH-a), which induces reversible ovarian shutdown in premenopausal women, was given to 10 women with moderate to severe PMS. Conjugated equine estrogen and medroxyprogesterone acetate were added. During treatment, all symptoms decreased significantly compared with baseline and placebo. Women using ERT with or without progesterone had better mood scores than those who did not. This work suggests that exogenous HRT will not necessarily cause PMS to return.

Summary

Some biological evidence supports a role of estrogen in cognitive function. The data thus far are inconclusive with respect to Alzheimer's disease and estrogen. Women treated with HRT for hot flashes may perform better than women not using HRT on cognitive function tests because of better sleep patterns rather than a direct neurological effect. These findings may be a direct estrogen effect as a result of alleviation of other distressing symptoms or a selection bias in the retrospective studies available. Only anecdotal evidence supports HRT in the etiology of depressive symptoms. Although estrogen is not an effective treatment for clinical depression, it may result in an improved sense of well-being in some women. At least two randomized, controlled trials showed that HRT does not induce or exacerbate PMS.

Osteoporosis

Because bone mass is highly correlated with bone strength, women with low bone mass are more likely than women with greater bone mass to have significant injury with minor trauma and, hence, the increased incidence of fractures. However, the absolute risk is still relatively low and quite variable (Cummings et al. 1993).

An average 50-year-old white woman in North America has approximately a 16%–17% lifetime risk of fracturing her hip (Cummings et al. 1993). Osteoporotic fracture rates increase exponentially with age in both men and women. At any given age, women have about double the risk of osteoporosis compared with that of men. This difference is partially explained by the difference in the peak bone mass between the sexes, bone loss associated with menopause, and the greater incidence of falling in older women. HRT is estimated to decrease the risk of osteoporosis by 30%–60% (see Chapter 6; Cauley et al. 1995).

Efficacy of Treatment

ERT with both oral and transdermal estrogen has been shown unequivocally at least to reduce the rate of bone loss and probably to maintain it (Barlow 1993; Lindsay and Tohme 1990). However, some women (probably fewer than 10%) (R. Josse, personal communication, November 1995) lose bone mass during HRT despite adequate compliance. This loss may represent other causes of osteoporosis in this group and not simply a lack of efficacy of HRT. Current users who started taking estrogen within 5 years of menopause are at decreased risk for hip, wrist, and all nonspinal fractures when compared with women who have never used estrogen (Cauley et al. 1995). There does not appear to be any significant difference in treatment or prevention of osteoporosis between oral and transdermal estrogen or between natural and synthetic estrogen when doses are equivalent (Grey et al. 1994). Although there are more long-term data with conjugated equine estrogens, the shorter-term data available with other estrogen preparations show equal efficacy. There is no single estrogen that is superior for the treatment or prevention of osteoporosis.

Progestins have a beneficial effect on bone independent of the effect of estrogen. Some preliminary data suggest that the scheduling of the progestin (cyclical versus continuous) may affect the bone density, but insufficient human evidence exists at present to guide clinical decisions. Currently, the combination of estrogen and progestin is probably the best alternative. Ongoing research may lead to increased enthusiasm for estrogen and androgen, but this option has not yet met with widespread support (Watts et al. 1995).

Duration

The rate of bone loss is greatest in the immediate postmenopausal period, probably within the first 2 years (Reid et al. 1994). Thus, the effect of HRT on the rate of bone loss is also greatest in this period. This finding has led to the interpretation that the benefits of estrogen are significant only in the first few years postmenopause, although this is not necessarily the case. The initial bone loss in this period is unlikely to be completely corrected with the addition of estrogen later on. However, any time that estrogen is added will result in a beneficial effect on bone density. In older women, the relative benefits of estrogen may be the same as those in younger women, but because the baseline rate of loss (i.e., percent change over time) is less, the absolute changes will not be as great. It may even be advantageous to offer treatment only to "older" postmenopausal women, because the prevalence of low bone density (i.e., osteoporosis) is greater in this age group, and the rate of occurrence of fractures is directly related to the bone density.

The benefit of HRT is thought to persist throughout a woman's life. Thus, there are theoretical reasons for using HRT indefinitely, but this is unlikely to be practical for most women. Once the estrogen is stopped, bone loss will begin at the rate of that of early menopause. Multiple bone density measurements can be used to predict when the bone mass will reach 1 or 2 standard deviations from the norm. HRT for the purpose of prevention of osteoporosis should be stopped as soon as this level is greater than the life expectancy of the woman. For example, based on the bone mass and the rate of bone loss, if a 60-year-old woman is expected to have bone density such that her risk of fracture would be relatively low at age 90, she may choose to discontinue HRT. This would be advantageous with respect to her risk of breast cancer, which appears to increase with increasing duration of use. If her bone mass was such that she would be at risk for a fracture within a very short time of discontinuing HRT, she may choose to continue HRT indefinitely.

Nonhormonal Treatment

Exercise. Although high-intensity strength-training exercises increase bone mineral, the increase is much less than that normally seen with HRT (<1%) (Nelson et al. 1994; Preisinger et al. 1995). However, exercise can result in a significant improvement over nothing at all. Poor compliance with regular physical activities is a major cause of the lack of effect of exercise in the prevention of osteoporosis. It is unknown whether estrogen and exercise have an additive effect. It is likely that the two are complementary, in reducing both osteoporosis and cardiovascular disease.

Diet. Adequate dietary calcium is essential to maintain bone mass. In women with inadequate dietary calcium, the addition of calcium will retard bone loss, however, again, to a lesser extent than HRT does (Looker et al. 1993; Reid et al. 1995). The risk of hip fracture appears to be lower in women with good calcium intake (Elders et al. 1994). Another contributor to bone mass is body fat. Body fat increases with menopause, independent of HRT use (Aloia et al. 1995). An overweight woman stresses her bones daily by the extra weight she carries and thus strengthens her bones.

Cardiovascular Disease

Cardiovascular disease is the leading cause of death in post-menopausal women (see also Chapter 6). At least one-third of all deaths in women in the United States are attributable to cardiovascular disease. Several lines of evidence suggest that estrogen is an important determinant of cardiovascular risk in women. Epidemiological data document low rates of coronary heart disease (CHD) in premenopausal women, a narrowing of the gender gap in CHD mortality after menopause, and elevated risk of CHD among young women with bilateral oophorectomy not treated with estrogen.

Efficacy of Treatment

The most obvious effect of estrogen with respect to cardiovascular disease is the change in lipid profile (Manson 1994; Psaty et al. 1993). An increase in high-density lipoproteins and a decrease in low-density lipoproteins result in approximately an 8%–12% improvement in the lipid profile (The Writing Group for the PEPI Trial 1995). These effects are attenuated but not completely obliterated with progestin. The protection afforded by postmenopausal ERT against cardiovascular disease is not fully explained by changes in plasma lipoproteins. A change in vascular reactivity also occurs with HRT (Collins et al. 1995; Gangar et al. 1991).

Regimen Selection

Observational studies have suggested that unopposed estrogens reduce the incidence of CHD in postmenopausal women, but little research has been done on the effect of combined therapy with estrogens and progestins, a regimen adopted in recent years to minimize the risk of endometrial hyperplasia and cancer. In clinical trials, the addition of progestins had an adverse effect on serum lipid levels, and these lipid effects have raised the question of whether combined estrogen-progestin therapy increases the risk of CHD as compared with the use of estrogen alone. Observational data suggest that nonusers of hormones, users of estrogens alone, or users of combined estrogen-progestin therapy appear to have a similar risk ratio for myocardial infarction. In summary, although laboratory evidence may suggest an adverse effect of adding progestins, this has not been borne out by epidemiological evidence. Furthermore, much of the original work has included progestins, such as norethindrone, a 19-nortestosterone derivative, which is in many ways pharmacologically different from medroxyprogesterone acetate and newer drugs such as oral micronized progesterone.

Elevated levels of endogenous testosterone in premenopausal women increase the risk of cardiovascular disease. This increased risk also appears to be true, although to a lesser extent, in post-menopausal women who have elevated levels of endogenous androgens but is not necessarily true in those with elevated levels of exogenous androgens (Sands and Studd 1995). Compared with the group treated with estrogen alone, in the estrogen-androgen-treated group, cholesterol, high-density lipoprotein cholesterol, and triglyceride levels decreased significantly. This lipoprotein effect has been confirmed by some, but not all, studies.

Duration

The beneficial effect of estrogen on lipids is not related to time since menopause, although the effect of estrogen on the peripheral vascular system may vary with time because the likelihood of atheromatous changes is greater with increasing age. Thus, in older women, estrogen would be more effective in secondary prevention of disease, and in younger postmenopausal women, estrogen would be more effective in primary prevention. Women with a new diagnosis of cardiovascular disease are being offered estrogen regardless of the number of years since menopause.

As with treatment of osteoporosis, treatment of cardiovascular disease should be discontinued when the risk of the disease is less than the risk of side effects of the treatment or when the risk of the disease is no longer clinically relevant. This may occur in very elderly women or in the presence of more imminent medical problems. It is unknown to what degree the beneficial effects of HRT persist after discontinuation. Even though the beneficial lipid changes would not persist, the woman would have benefited by the lack of progression of atherosclerosis during the years she was taking HRT.

For a discussion of genitourinary and sexual symptoms, please refer to Chapters 2, 5, and 6 in this volume. Irregular menstrual bleeding is discussed thoroughly in Chapter 2.

Risks of Hormone Replacement Therapy

Despite the beneficial effects of HRT, many women are reluctant to consider HRT because of the potential for risk of, primarily, breast cancer. More women are concerned about breast cancer than about cardiovascular disease. From a policy-making perspective, even if HRT did increase the relative risk of breast cancer (e.g., an increase of even 50%), it would still result in an absolute decrease in deaths because of the lives saved by the reduction in heart disease.

Breast Cancer

The rate of breast cancer cases has increased steadily since 1950, with a sharp rise in the 1980s (Garfinkel et al. 1994). The increased incidence of breast cancer coincides with an increased use of mammography in asymptomatic women in the 1980s. One explanation for the apparent rise in breast cancer in women taking HRT is a screening bias (Seeley 1994). Women using HRT are more likely to have mammograms and are thus more likely to have breast cancer diagnosed.

The largest study of HRT and breast cancer risk is that of Colditz et al. (1995) and the Nurses Health Study (see also Chapter 6). The study suggested an elevated risk of invasive breast cancer among postmenopausal women who were currently taking estrogen alone or combined estrogen and progestin. The increase in risk was most pronounced among women older than 55 and was largely limited to the women who had used HRT for 5 years or longer. Compared with other women in the same region, the women taking estrogen had an overall relative risk of breast cancer of 1.1. The relative risk increased with the duration of estrogen treatment, reaching 1.7 after 9 years (confidence interval 1.1–2.7).

Only one randomized, prospective clinical study is attempting to define the influence, if any, of ERT on the clinical course of breast cancer (Vassilopoulou-Sellin and Theriault 1994). Women with stage I or stage II breast cancer and no evidence of breast cancer disease for at least 2 years were randomized to receive ERT (conjugated estrogens 0.625 mg, days 1–25) or no intervention (control). Approximately 30% of women with a history of breast cancer declined participation because of a fear of cancer, whereas 30% either have already decided to take ERT or are willing to participate in the study (Vassilopoulou-Sellin and Klein 1996). No preliminary results are available at this time. Hormone-sensitive tumors, such as breast cancer, are currently considered an absolute contraindication to HRT. Patients who develop breast cancer during HRT have fewer locally advanced cancers (large tumors and extensive lymph node involvement) and more well-differentiated cancers (infiltrating lobular cancers and grade 1 cancer) compared with patients not using HRT who develop breast cancer. However, the number of patients with estradiol or progesterone receptors was lower in the hormone-treated group. This is often thought to signal a long-term poorer outcome. Nevertheless, metastasis-free survival curves showed a tendency for better prognosis in hormone-treated patients in one study (Bonnier et al. 1995).

The aggregate experience of HRT is highly suggestive of an increased risk of breast cancer. The clinically meaningful risk has yet to be determined. This will be based on the balance of the risks and benefits of HRT to other organs and overall health. It will also be patient specific with respect to her fear of cancer. Paradoxically, there is new enthusiasm for the use of HRT in patients with breast cancer because of the appreciation of diminution of the quality of life in women with hot flashes. Some women with breast cancer are so distressed by hot flashes that they are willing to risk exacerbation of the hormone-sensitive tumors to alleviate their symptoms.

Duration

There is no consensus as to when to stop HRT. Because the risks of breast cancer appear to increase with increasing duration of HRT, it would seem prudent to continue for no more than 10 or 15 years, or until age 70.

Endometrial Cancer

Endometrial cancer is always a concern in any woman experiencing postmenopausal bleeding, especially those exposed to estrogen alone. In a meta-analysis of 10 studies, unopposed estrogen use for 5 years or longer was associated with a large increase in the risk of endometrial cancer. In terms of absolute risk, endometrial hyperplasia develops in approximately 20% of women treated with estrogen alone and in <1% for any treatment that includes acetate (Woodruff and Pickar 1994). In terms of relative risk, unopposed estrogen increases one's risk of endometrial cancer approximately eightfold. Approximately 40% of cases of endometrial hyperplasia will progress to frank malignancy. Use for shorter duration also increases risk; however, among women who used estrogens for less than 6 months, any increased risk that may exist appears to be very small. Risk appears to decrease with increasing time since cessation of use but does not completely disappear. Most of the studies found no differences between oral synthetic estrogens and conjugated estrogens with respect to cancer risk; none found a difference between cyclic and continuous regimens.

An increased risk of endometrial cancer can be avoided by the use of progestins (Gambrell 1986; see also Chapters 2 and 6). Endometrial cancer is a risk only in women who choose not to take progestins, which is often because of the side effects (discussed later in this chapter). The risk can also be minimized by adequate screening for endometrial hyperplasia. Vaginal ultrasound for measuring endometrial thickness can be a sensitive technique for diagnosing endometrial disease (Dorum et al. 1993). Several studies have shown that an endometrial thickness of 4 mm or less has a low risk for endometrial carcinoma. The sensitivity and the negative predictive value of vaginal ultrasound are not high enough to replace histological examination of the endometrium, but ultrasound is a simple and a noninvasive diagnostic method that can identify women at high risk for endometrial cancer (Nasri et al. 1991).

Thromboembolic Risk

The risk of estrogen-mediated thrombotic episodes is estrogen dose dependent. Thrombophlebitis has not been reported in controlled trials of HRT. The concerns raised with oral contraceptives do not apply to HRT. It is helpful to remember that 5 mg of ethinyl estradiol is equivalent to 0.625 mg of conjugated equine estrogens. Most low-dose birth control pills contain 30 mg of ethinyl estradiol. No studies have examined the specific relationship between HRT and deep venous thrombosis, although many have implicated oral contraceptives. Therefore, even patients with a history of thromboembolism in pregnancy or associated with oral contraceptive use should be offered physiological HRT after complete examination. Furthermore, studies of deep venous thrombosis that identify gender suggested that there is no gender difference in deep venous thrombosis or pulmonary embolism in the elderly (Kniffen et al. 1994; Quinn et al. 1992).

Special Considerations

Table 7–3 lists the standard contraindications to HRT. Some liver tumors are estrogen sensitive and would be considered a contraindication to HRT; however, in many other conditions, HRT is acceptable, particularly if transdermal estrogens, which are not metabolized by the liver, are used. Despite evidence to the contrary, gallbladder disease is still considered by some to be a relative contraindication to HRT (LaVecchia et al. 1992; Mohr et al. 1991).

Summary

The change in risk of CHD, hip fracture, stroke, and breast cancer with HRT is summarized in Table 7–4.

Table 7–3.   Contraindications to hormone replacement therapy

Absolute contraindications
  Unexplained vaginal bleeding prior to investigation
  Active liver disease
  Breast cancer
  Active vascular thrombosis

Relative contraindications
  Migraine headaches
  History of thromboembolism
  Familial hypertriglyceridemia
  Uterine leiomyomas
  Endometriosis
  Gallbladder disease
  Uterine cancer
  Chronic hepatic dysfunction

Table 7–4. Change in risk of disease with hormone replacement therapy

Condition	Relative risk with estrogen compared with no treatment	Relative risk with estrogen-progestin compared with no treatment
Coronary heart disease	0.65	0.65–8.0
Stroke	0.75	0.75
Hip fracture	0.90	0.85
Breast cancer	1.25	1.25–5.0

Troubleshooting With Hormone Replacement Therapy

Reasons for Discontinuation of Hormonal Treatment

Troublesome side effects related to HRT are caused by either estrogen effects, progestin effects, or a combination of the two. Vaginal bleeding with HRT is a common reason given by women for nonadherence to hormonal treatment.

Estrogen Effects

Estrogen effects are usually dose related but are often idiosyncratic. Breast tenderness is a common complaint, particularly in women who were hypoestrogenic for a significant period before starting HRT. The dose can be lowered, but it must be remembered that the effects of estrogen on the cardiovascular system and bone are dose related. Reducing the estrogen dose too much may negate the beneficial effects (Marsh et al. 1994).

Some women appear to be more sensitive to some types of estrogen. Trying other products is worthwhile. Transdermal preparations deliver a more even dose and may be beneficial for some women, particularly those with estrogen-sensitive headaches.

Progestin Effects

Progestin effects are usually the most bothersome to women. These effects include bloating, headaches, irregular bleeding, and probably mood changes. These symptoms are best treated by switching to a continuous combined regimen. This regimen has the dual benefit of minimizing the daily dose and reducing the fluctuations as experienced in the cyclic regimen. The newer progestins, such as oral micronized progesterone, are advertised as having fewer side effects than older progestins, but this has not yet been proven in clinical practice. For women who cannot tolerate the progestin effects, unopposed estrogen can be considered. The clinician must explain the risk of endometrial hyperplasia and malignancy, and the patient must be able to commit to close follow-up with at least biyearly transvaginal ultrasound.

Vaginal Bleeding

Vaginal bleeding with HRT is most likely to be uterine in origin. However, it is important to remember that bleeding can also occur from the vagina, cervix, and, very rarely, the fallopian tube. Therefore, a full gynecological examination is mandatory.

Uterine bleeding in a woman receiving HRT may be a result of either preexisting anatomical abnormalities or hormonal manipulation. Investigations should include documentation of the presence or absence of uterine polyps and intramural fibroids. Ultrasound (either transvaginal or abdominal) can be used for this examination. In addition, hysterosonography (ultrasound in conjunction with the instillation of a distending media to better outline endometrial contour) is becoming more widely used. If necessary, diagnostic hysteroscopy with either local or general anesthesia may be used to visualize the uterine cavity directly.

If no anatomical abnormality is found, bleeding as a direct result of HRT must be considered. Tissue diagnosis is essential. Outpatient endometrial biopsy has replaced diagnostic dilatation and curettage as the test of choice. Any malignant or premalignant changes would mandate a change in treatment. If the woman had been taking ERT, the addition of progestin may suffice. The detailed management of endometrial neoplasia is beyond the scope of this chapter.

In women with irregular bleeding while taking estrogen and cyclic progestin, treatment changes may include switching to a con-

tinuous regimen, altering either the dose or the duration of progestin, or altering the dose or type of estrogen. Typically, women
who experience bleeding before the completion of their 5-mg
course of progestin require a higher dose. Bleeding while using a
continuous regimen usually abates with time, as the endometrium
becomes more atrophic. If this does not occur, women may choose
to revert to a cyclic regimen. This regimen is associated with bleeding but will provide a regular, predictable schedule of bleeding,
which may be preferable to the irregular spotting associated with
the continuous regimen.

The idiosyncratic response to HRT cannot be overemphasized.
This is as true for the endometrial response as for the cognitive or
mood responses. Finding an acceptable regimen that alleviates distressing bleeding may be a slow, iterative process that involves
repeated refinements of the therapy, which cannot always be
anticipated.

Summary

The management of menopause should be based on the preferences of the individual patient rather than on symptom severity
alone. Thus, the fear of breast cancer is as significant to the decision-making process as is the actual statistical risk. The challenge
for the clinician and woman is to determine which outcome may
need to be compromised in order to maximize another. The uncertainty of the information available at this time, the nonmedical component of the issues, and the potential side effects of the therapy
make the decision about HRT one of the most formidable tasks for
middle-aged women today.

References

Abraham S, Perz J, Clarkson R, et al: Australian women's perceptions of
    HRT over 10 years. Maturitas 21:91–95, 1995
Aloia JF, Vaswani A, Russo L, et al: The influence of menopause and hor-
    monal replacement therapy on body cell mass and body fat mass. Am
    J Obstet Gynecol 172:896–900, 1995
Barlow DH: HRT and osteoporosis. Clin Rheumatol 7:535–548, 1993

Barrett-Connor E, Kritz-Silverstein D: Estrogen replacement therapy and cognitive function in older women. JAMA 269:2637–2641, 1993

Bonnier P, Romain S, Giacalone PL, et al: Clinical and biologic prognostic factors in breast cancer diagnosed during postmenopausal HRT. Obstet Gynecol 85:11–17, 1995

Brenner DE, Kukull WA, Stergachis A, et al: Postmenopausal estrogen replacement therapy and the risk of Alzheimer's disease: a population-based case-control study. Am J Epidemiol 140:262–267, 1994

Campbell-Brown M, McEwan HP: Scottish gynaecologists: their views on HRT. Health Bull (Edinb) 50:248–251, 1992

Cano A: Compliance to HRT in menopausal women controlled in a third level academic centre. Maturitas 20:91–99, 1994

Cauley JA, Seeley DG, Ensrud K, et al: Estrogen replacement therapy and fractures in older women: Study of Osteoporotic Fractures Research Group. Ann Intern Med 122:9–16, 1995

Cheung AP, Wren BG: A cost-effectiveness analysis of HRT in the menopause. Med J Aust 156:312–316, 1992

Colditz GA, Hankinson SE, Hunter DJ, et al: The use of estrogen and progestin and the risk of breast cancer in postmenopausal women. N Engl J Med 332:1589–1593, 1995

Collins P, Rosano GM, Sarrel PM, et al: 17 beta-estradiol attenuates acetylcholine-induced coronary arterial constriction in women but not men with coronary heart disease. Circulation 92:24–30, 1995

Cummings SR, Black DM, Nevitt MC, et al: Bone density at various sites for prediction of hip fracture. Lancet 341:72–75, 1993

Daly E, Gray A, Barlow D, et al: Measuring the impact of menopausal symptoms on quality of life. BMJ 307:836–840, 1993

Dorum A, Kristensen GB, Langebrekke A, et al: Evaluation of endometrial thickness measured by endovaginal ultrasound in women with postmenopausal bleeding. Acta Obstet Gynecol Scand 72:116–119, 1993

Elders PJ, Lips P, Netelenbos JC, et al: Long-term effect of calcium supplementation on bone loss in perimenopausal women. J Bone Miner Res 9:963–970, 1994

Elstein AS, Holzman GB, Ravitch MM, et al: Comparison of physicians' decision regarding estrogen replacement therapy for menopausal women and decisions derived from a decision analytic model. Am J Med 80:246–256, 1986

Foster GV, Zacur HA, Rock JA: Hot flashes in postmenopausal women ameliorated by danazol. Fertil Steril 43:401–404, 1985

Gambrell RD Jr: Prevention of endometrial cancer with progestogens. Maturitas 8:159–168, 1986

Gangar KF, Vyas S, Whitehead M, et al: Pulsatility index in internal carotid artery in relation to transdermal oestradiol and time since menopause. Lancet 338:839–842, 1991

Garfinkel L, Boring CC, Heath CW Jr: Changing trends: an overview of breast cancer incidence and mortality. Cancer 74:222–227, 1994

Goldberg RM, Loprinzi CL, O'Fallon JR, et al: Transdermal clonidine for ameliorating tamoxifen-induced hot flashes. J Clin Oncol 12:155–158, 1994

Grady D, Rubin SM, Petitti DB, et al: Hormone therapy to prevent disease and prolong life in postmenopausal women. Ann Intern Med 117:1016–1037, 1992

Grey AB, Cundy TF, Reid IR: Continuous combined oestrogen/progestin therapy is well tolerated and increases bone density at the hip and spine in post-menopausal osteoporosis. Clin Endocrinol (Oxf) 40:671–677, 1994

Hammond CB: Women's concerns with HRT—compliance issues. Fertil Steril 62:157S–160S, 1994

Henderson VW, Paganini-Hill A, Emanuel CK, et al: Estrogen replacement therapy in older women: comparisons between Alzheimer's disease cases and non-demented control subjects. Arch Neurol 51:896–900, 1994

Hunter MS, Liao KL: Intentions to use HRT in a community sample of 45-year-old women. Maturitas 20:13–23, 1994

Kampen DL, Sherwin BB: Estrogen use and verbal memory in healthy postmenopausal women. Obstet Gynecol 83:979–983, 1994

Kirkham C, Hahn PM, Van Vugt DA, et al: A randomized, double-blind, placebo-controlled, cross-over trial to assess the side effects of medroxyprogesterone acetate in HRT. Obstet Gynecol 78:93–97, 1991

Kniffin WD Jr, Baron JA, Barrett J, et al: The epidemiology of diagnosed pulmonary embolism and deep venous thrombosis in the elderly. Arch Intern Med 154:861–866, 1994

LaVecchia C, Negri E, D'Avanzo B, et al: Oral contraceptives and non-contraceptive oestrogens in the risk of gallstone disease requiring surgery. J Epidemiol Community Health 46:234–236, 1992

Limouzin-Lamothe MA, Mairon N, Joyce CR, et al: Quality of life after the menopause: influence of hormonal replacement therapy. Am J Obstet Gynecol 170:618–624, 1994

Lindsay R, Tohme JF: Estrogen treatment of patients with established post-menopausal osteoporosis. Obstet Gynecol 76:290–295, 1990

Looker AC, Harris TB, Madans JH, et al: Dietary calcium and hip fracture risk: the NHANES I Epidemiologic Follow-Up Study. Osteoporos Int 3:177–184, 1993

Manson J: Menopausal HRT and atherosclerotic disease. Am Heart J 129:1337–1343, 1994

Marsh MS, Whitcroft S, Whitehead MI: Paradoxical effects of HRT on breast tenderness in postmenopausal women. Maturitas 19:97–102, 1994

Mezrow G, Shoupe D, Spicer D, et al: Depot leuprolide acetate with estrogen and progestin add-back for long-term treatment of premenstrual syndrome. Fertil Steril 62:932–937, 1994

Mohr GC, Kritz-Silverstein D, Barrett-Connor E: Plasma lipids and gallbladder disease. Am J Epidemiol 134:78–85, 1991

Nasri MN, Shepherd JH, Setchell ME, et al: The role of vaginal scan in measurement of endometrial thickness in postmenopausal women. Br J Obstet Gynaecol 98:470–475, 1991

Nelson ME, Fiatarone MA, Morganti CM, et al: Effects of high-intensity strength training on multiple risk factors for osteoporotic fractures: a randomized controlled trial. JAMA 272:1909–1914, 1994

Paganini-Hill A, Henderson VW: Estrogen deficiency and Alzheimer disease. Am J Epidemiol 140:256–261, 1994

Palinkas LA, Barrett-Connor E: Estrogen use and depressive symptoms in postmenopausal women. Obstet Gynecol 80:30–36, 1992

Place VA, Powers M, Darley PE, et al: A double-blind comparative study of Estraderm and Premarin in the amelioration of postmenopausal symptoms. Am J Obstet Gynecol 152:1092–1099, 1985

Preisinger E, Alacamlioglu Y, Pils K, et al: Therapeutic exercise in the prevention of bone loss: a controlled trial with women after menopause. Am J Phys Med Rehabil 74:120–123, 1995

Psaty BM, Heckbert SR, Atkins D, et al: The use of myocardial infarction associated with combined use of estrogen, progestin in postmenopausal women. Arch Intern Med 153:1421–1427, 1993

Quinn DA, Thompson BT, Terrin ML, et al: A prospective investigation of pulmonary embolism in women and men. JAMA 268:1689–1696, 1992

Reid IR, Ames RW, Evans MC, et al: Determinants of the rate of bone loss in normal postmenopausal women. J Clin Endocrinol Metab 79:950–954, 1994

Reid IR, Ames RW, Evans MC, et al: Long-term effects of calcium supplementation on bone loss and fractures in postmenopausal women: a randomized controlled trial. Am J Med 98:331–335, 1995

Roberts PJ: Reported satisfaction among women receiving HRT in a dedicated general practice clinic and in a normal consultation. Br J Gen Pract 45:79–81, 1995

Sands R, Studd J: Exogenous androgens on post menopausal women. Am J Med 98:76S–79S, 1995

Seeley T: Do women taking HRT have a higher uptake of screening mammograms? Maturitas 19:93–96, 1994

Sherwin BB, Gelfand MM, Brender W: Androgen enhances sexual motivation in females: a prospective, crossover study of sex steroid administration in the surgical menopause. Psychosom Med 47:339–351, 1985

Steingold KA, Laufer L, Chetkowski RJ, et al: Treatment of hot flashes with transdermal estradiol administration. J Clin Endocrinol Metab 61:627–632, 1985

Swartzman LC, Edelberg R, Kemmann E: Impact of stress on objectively recorded menopausal hot flushes and on flush report bias. Health Psychol 9:529–545, 1990

Thompson W: Estrogen replacement therapy in practice: trends and issues. Am J Obstet Gynecol 173:990–993, 1995

Tosteson AN, Rosenthal DI, Melton LJ III, et al: Cost effectiveness of screening perimenopausal white women for osteoporosis: bone densitometry and HRT. Ann Intern Med 113:594–603, 1990

Vassilopoulou-Sellin R, Klein MJ: ERT after treatment for localized breast carcinoma: patient reponses and opinion. Cancer 78:1043–1048, 1996

Vassilopoulou-Sellin R, Theriault RL: Randomized prospective trial of estrogen-replacement therapy in women with a history of breast cancer: Monogr Natl Cancer Inst 16:153–159, 1994

Watts NB, Notelovitz M, Timmons MC, et al: Comparison of oral estrogens and estrogens plus androgen on bone mineral density, menopausal symptoms, and lipid-lipoprotein profiles in surgical menopause. Obstet Gynecol 85:529–537, 1995

Woodruff JD, Pickar JH: Incidence of endometrial hyperplasia in postmenopausal women taking conjugated estrogens (Premarin) with medroxyprogesterone acetate or conjugated estrogens alone: the Menopause Study Group. Am J Obstet Gynecol 170:1213–1223, 1994

The Writing Group for the PEPI Trial: Effects of estrogen or estrogen/progestin regimens on heart disease risk factors in postmenopausal women: the Postmenopausal Estrogen/Progestin Interventions (PEPI) Trial. JAMA 273:199–208, 1995

Wysowski DK, Golden L, Burke L: Use of menopausal estrogens and medroxyprogesterone in the United States, 1982–1992. Obstet Gynecol 85:6–10, 1995

CHAPTER 8

Psychiatric Aspects

Dara A. Charney, M.D., F.R.C.P.C.
Donna E. Stewart, M.D., F.R.C.P.C.

Although all women of a certain age experience menopause, not all women report unpleasant symptoms during menopause. Menopause is not a disorder, but the changes that occur in menopause may result in significant psychic and/or somatic distress in some women. Although it is important for health care professionals not to characterize menopause as a disease state, it is equally valuable for practitioners to understand its putative etiological role in those women who have clinical symptoms during menopause. In this chapter, we discuss the psychiatric literature, symptoms, etiological models, clinical examples, and general treatment recommendations for women who have psychiatric disorders during menopause.

Psychiatric Literature on Menopause

The relation of psychological symptoms to the occurrence of menopause is controversial. Psychiatric research on menopause is often contradictory, partially because of significant methodological inconsistencies in the literature. For example, some studies use community samples of women, whereas others use clinical samples. Some investigators inappropriately extrapolate from clinic populations to the general population and tend to overly pathologize the experience of menopause, whereas other researchers falsely equate the experiences of the general population to those of a symptomatic subpopulation of women who require medical and/or psychological interventions.

Further difficulty arises from variable inclusion criteria. Some studies include both naturally and surgically menopausal women; the latter tend to have poorer health, experience more depression and somatic symptoms, and use more health services both before and after their surgery (J. B. McKinlay et al. 1987). The failure to separate these two groups of women may falsely elevate the rates of psychiatric disorders among all women.

Other limitations of the menopause literature result from ambiguous terminology. In particular, most studies define menopause status by age or by termination of menses rather than by more accurate measurements of gonadal hormone levels. Many women in perimenopause have postmenopausal levels of estrogen and progesterone (Schmidt and Rubinow 1991). Furthermore, the decline of ovarian function in perimenopause may have more pronounced psychoendocrine effects than the cessation of ovarian function at menopause. There are also problems with the definition of clinically significant symptoms. Most research relies on self-report symptom data, without measurements of impairment, severity, or pervasiveness and without clinical interviews. Symptoms are multidetermined and do not necessarily reflect clinically verifiable psychiatric syndromes.

Psychiatric Symptoms Attributed to Menopause

The concept of involutional melancholia was introduced by Kraepelin in 1896. He distinguished it from manic-depressive illness and other forms of psychosis. The clinical presentation he described included an agitated depression with hypochondriac or nihilistic delusions, a particularly rigid or obsessive personality, no prior episodes of depression or mania, and a variable outcome. More recent studies have not supported the validity of the involutional melancholia construct. There is no symptom pattern specific to depression that occurs during menopause, as compared with depression that occurs at other times in adult life (Weissman 1979), the rate of psychiatric hospitalization during menopause is not elevated (Winokur 1973), and the prevalence of major depression probably is not increased in the postmenopausal years (Hällström and Samuelsson 1985; Schmidt and Rubinow 1991). Accordingly, involutional melancholia was subsumed under the broader classification of major depression in DSM-III (American Psychiatric Association 1980).

Other forms of psychological distress may be associated with menopause (see also Gise, Chapter 3, in this volume). In particular, there may be a clinical picture of atypical depression or neurasthenia during menopause (Schmidt and Rubinow 1991). Perimenopausal women attending menopause clinics also may have significant anxiety symptoms (e.g., nervousness, fearfulness, tenseness, panic, and restlessness) (Stewart et al. 1992).

Neugarten and Kraines (1965) conducted one of the first surveys of menopause symptomatology. They questioned 460 American women between ages 13 and 64 and identified two peaks of psychic and somatic distress: one at puberty and the other at menopause. These "menopausal" women had elevated rates of depression, irritability, nervousness, headache, and other somatic symptoms. Several subsequent studies examined the prevalence of emotional and behavioral disturbances in larger samples of middle-aged women. Jaszmann et al. (1969) surveyed 3,000 Dutch women between ages 40 and 60 and found that complaints of "mental imbalance," irritability, fatigue, headache, and dizziness were more common in women with irregular menses who were considered to be perimenopausal. Bungay et al. (1980) reported a peak of "minor mental symptoms" among 1,120 British women immediately prior to the mean age at menopause. Other researchers demonstrated similarly elevated levels of psychological distress in perimenopausal women, by using substantially different methodology, including standardized clinical interviews (Ballinger 1975).

Although a number of studies have reported an increased prevalence of depressive, anxiety, and other psychological symptoms during menopause, several studies of large nonclinical populations have yielded contradictory results (Kaufert 1980; S. M. McKinlay and Jeffreys 1974; S. M. McKinlay and McKinlay

1985; Thompson et al. 1973). J. B. McKinlay et al. (1987) prospectively studied 2,500 women between ages 45 and 55 and found no association between the onset of menopause and clinically significant depressive symptoms. In this sample, the most marked increases in depression occurred in surgically menopausal women and in women with multiple work- and family-related stressors.

Greene and Cooke's (1980) survey of Scottish women also indicated that increased psychic and somatic distress in perimenopause was directly correlated with a high degree of life stress; neither age nor menopausal status accounted for a significant portion of the variance. Hunter et al. (1986) used a multiple regression analysis to determine whether menopausal status was associated with symptom occurrence. They found that vasomotor symptoms and sexual difficulties were best predicted by menopausal status, whereas depression was best predicted by social class but also was influenced by menopausal status.

Thus, menopause does not appear to be characterized by an excess of clinically significant emotional or behavioral disorders nor is there a specific menopause-related psychiatric syndrome. In contrast, minor depressive, anxiety, and psychosomatic symptoms seem to be more frequent in perimenopause; in studies of women seeking treatment for physical symptoms related to menopause, many perimenopausal women report psychological distress (Stewart et al. 1992). For those women who do experience psychological distress in this context, the etiology of these symptoms remains unclear.

Overview of Various Etiological Models

There are several competing etiological theories of the occurrence of psychological symptoms in some menopausal women (Ballinger 1990; Dennerstein and Burrows 1978; see also Baram, Gise, Mogul, and Shapiro, Chapters 2, 3, 6, and 7, respectively, in this volume). A psychoendocrine hypothesis points toward the relationship between decreasing levels of gonadal hormones and depressed affect (Sherwin 1994). Other biological models view these symptoms as secondary manifestations of disabling vasomotor symptoms (Campbell 1976) or as consequences of increasing chronological age

(Leidy 1994; see also Baram, Mogul, and Feldman and Netz, Chapters 2, 6, and 12, respectively, in this volume).

Psychosocial theories (see Chapter 3) emphasize life stressors that occur at about the same time as menopause: children leaving home and an "empty nest," possible poor health and death of parents and in-laws, altered family roles, and a changing social support network (Cooke 1985; J. B. McKinlay et al. 1987). Psychoanalytic models suggest that the heavy investment in fertility and procreation leads some women to become depressed at the inevitable loss of these abilities in menopause (Deutsch 1945; see Stotland, Chapter 9, in this volume). Cross-cultural research has brought to light both sociocultural explanations (e.g., differences in social status and familial roles of women in middle age) and biocultural explanations (e.g., variations in genetics, fertility patterns, diet, and environment) of this phenomenon (Lock 1986; see also Weber, Chapter 4, in this volume).

Psychoendocrine Model

From an endocrine standpoint, menopause is characterized by elevated serum levels of luteinizing and follicle-stimulating hormones and reduced levels of circulating estrogens and progesterones (see Chapter 2). Decreases in gonadal hormones are not related in a simple or direct way to psychological distress during menopause. Sex steroid levels per se have failed to distinguish symptomatic from asymptomatic women, and specific hormonal abnormalities have not been found for peri- or postmenopausal depressions (Schmidt and Rubinow 1991). Therefore, abnormal levels of estrogen or progesterone do not trigger psychological symptoms during menopause; however, some women may have an increased vulnerability to normal hormonal changes associated with menopause.

If women who are depressed during menopause are indeed more sensitive to normal hormonal changes, then they may have been vulnerable to mood disturbances associated with other reproductive events. This hypothesis has been tested in the psychiatric literature in retrospective studies. In one study (Stewart and Boydell 1993), 259 consecutive menopausal women attending a menopause clinic were divided into highest (n = 42) and lowest (n = 44) psychological distress groups on the General Severity Index of the Brief Symptom Inventory (Derogatis and Spencer 1982). Subjects with the highest psychological distress during menopause were significantly more likely to report a psychiatric history, particularly depression, previous antidepressant treatment, dysphoria related to oral contraceptive use, postnatal blues, and postpartum depression, than were subjects with the lowest distress during menopause. Many factors (e.g., selective recall, halo effect, coping strategies) may account for these women reporting more affective symptoms during reproductive events, but these results may also reflect a subgroup of women who are vulnerable to normal gonadal hormonal changes as a trigger for affective syndromes.

O'Hara et al. (1991) similarly found that women with postnatal blues were more likely to have had previous depressions, including premenstrual and postpartum depressions, than women without postnatal blues. Warner et al. (1991) reported that women with late-luteal-phase dysphoric disorder had a higher incidence of depression and postpartum depression than did women in the general population. The evidence is suggestive of a subgroup of women who are vulnerable to affective syndromes at times of normal changes in the reproductive cycle. A longitudinal epidemiological study from menarche to menopause is needed to prospectively study these putative associations.

Several authors point to depression associated with various reproductive events to explain the greater lifetime prevalence of affective illness in women than men. Steiner (1992) postulated that the menstrual cycle may function as a biopsychosocial "zeitgeber," or time giver, and may be involved in the regulation or dysregulation of mood in women. In some women, this may contribute to female-specific mood disorders by triggering a cascade of events along the hypothalamic-pituitary-gonadal axis. Parry (1992) reviewed the association of affective symptoms with times of gonadal hormonal flux—menstruation, parturition, and menopause—and suggested that a model of conditioning, behavioral sensitization, and electrophysiological kindling is supported under the influence of reproductive hormones.

Case 1

Ms. A, a 53-year-old lawyer, presented with irritability, insomnia, anxiety, and mood lability. Her family life was generally happy, and her job offered many opportunities that she used to enjoy. Recently, she has felt tired and disinterested in work. She has a history of postnatal depression following the births of her two children, and, in recent years, she has experienced 1-week periods of profound sadness before menstruation. Her menstrual periods have become irregular and scant in the past year. She complained of hot flashes, night sweats, and palpitations. After Ms. A began taking an estrogen-progesterone oral regimen, the hot flashes, night sweats, palpitations, and insomnia greatly declined. However, she remained anxious and intermittently sad during the following 6 months. After having several weeks of moderately severe depressive symptoms, she returned to her physician. The physician prescribed a selective serotonin inhibitor (fluoxetine 20 mg/day), and Ms. A felt consistently better after a month of treatment. Ms. A and her physician agreed to continue antidepressant treatment for 6 months and to discontinue the fluoxetine if she maintained her improvement. Ms. A plans to continue taking her hormonal regimen indefinitely because she has a family history of osteoporosis, and her bone scan showed osteopenia.

Neurobiological Effects of Estrogen

The psychoendocrine hypothesis of a causal connection between gonadal hormonal changes and affective syndromes in some women is strengthened by evidence that sex steroids influence mood. Estrogen has both direct and inductive effects on neurons (Kelly et al. 1977; O'Malley and Means 1974). Estrogen receptors have been found on neurons in areas of the brain that are implicated in mood regulation (McEwen 1980), and several neurotransmitter systems may be responsive to gonadal hormones (McEwen et al. 1984). The most compelling data come from animal and human research on the complex relation between estrogen and serotonin. Serotonin deficiency is considered to be an important causal factor in depression. Several mechanisms by which estrogen can enhance serotonergic transmission have been described.

Estrogen results in an increased density of tritiated imipramine binding sites on platelets in rats (Kendall et al. 1981) and in oophorectomized women (Sherwin and Suranyi-Cadotte 1990). A decreased density of tritiated imipramine binding sites on platelets is regarded as a biological correlate of depression.

Estrogen displaces tryptophan, a precursor of serotonin, from its binding sites on plasma albumin (Alyward 1973), which results in an increased concentration of free tryptophan in the brain. A significant negative correlation between depression scores and free tryptophan levels was reported in oophorectomized women (Alyward 1976).

Estrogen increases the degradation of monoamine oxidase, the enzyme that catabolizes serotonin and other neurotransmitters, thereby increasing their brain concentrations and synaptic availability (Luine and McEwen 1977). In contrast, progesterone decreases the degradation of monoamine oxidase, thereby decreasing brain concentrations of neurotransmitters (Backstrom 1977).

Estrogen Clinical Trials and Mood

Clinical trials of gonadal hormones provide further evidence of the specific beneficial effects of estrogen on mood. In particular, physiological doses of estrogen improve mood in nonpsychiatric populations of symptomatic menopausal women (Dennerstein et al. 1979; Ditkoff et al. 1991; Montgomery et al. 1987; Sherwin 1988a; Sherwin and Gelfand 1985; Weisbader and Kurzrok 1983). This effect appears to be independent of the action of estrogen on concurrent hormone-sensitive physical symptoms, such as hot flashes (Campbell and Whitehead 1977).

In several of these studies (Dennerstein et al. 1979; Sherwin 1988a; Sherwin and Gelfand 1985), all women had undergone surgical menopause, and some women received unopposed estrogen. In women with an intact uterus, cyclic progesterones are necessary to counteract the endometrial proliferative action of estrogens. Women who are given estrogen plus progesterone may experience a dampening of mood compared with women who are given estrogen alone (Dennerstein et al. 1979; Holst et al. 1989). A prospective study of naturally menopausal women found that women who received high-dose estrogen with progesterone had more positive affect than those who received low-dose estrogen with progesterone (Sherwin 1991). Therefore, the depressive effects of progesterone may be attenuated by a higher estrogen-to-progesterone dose ratio.

Although these studies suggest that estrogen may enhance mood in a nonclinical menopausal population, evidence is lacking for estrogen as a treatment of clinical depression. In one study, women with severe, refractory depression responded to a 3-month course of pharmacological doses of conjugated estrogens (Premarin 15–25 mg/day) (Klaiber et al. 1979). However, this regimen is impractical because of the risks associated with such high doses. Estrogen used as an adjuvant to tricyclic antidepressants has had mixed results (Prange et al. 1976; Shapira et al. 1985; Stahl 1996). Methodological inconsistencies make these findings difficult to compare and interpret. Studies included both premenopausal and postmenopausal women, bipolar patients, and highly treatment-resistant patients (Prange et al. 1976; Shapira et al. 1985). The effectiveness of estrogen augmentation in depressed menopausal women has not yet been adequately tested, but early reports appear promising (Stahl 1996).

Estrogen Clinical Trials and Cognition

Sex steroids also may influence cognition (see also Chapters 6 and 7). Symptoms of impaired cognitive functioning, particularly memory, are common in menopausal women, both with and without concurrent symptoms of depression. Several early studies reported improvements in memory following estrogen replacement therapy (Campbell and Whitehead 1977; Schneider 1982); however, these findings were based solely on self-report data. More recently, Sherwin (1988b) examined surgically menopausal women and reported that those women who received estrogen maintained their memory and abstract reasoning scores postoperatively, whereas those who received placebo had lower scores. Another prospective study of oophorectomized women produced similar findings (Phillips and Sherwin 1992); estrogen therapy increased these women's scores on a paired-associations task and on immediate paragraph recall.

Sherwin (1994) suggested that estrogen seems to play a role in the maintenance of short-term memory in menopausal women, but the capacity for long-term memory does not appear to be influenced by the hormonal milieu.

Case 2

Ms. B, a 48-year-old homemaker, presented with sadness, irritability, insomnia, anxiety, and decreased concentration and memory. She felt more anxious and depressed in the mornings, cried daily, and often ruminated about her marriage and her future. As a result of her husband's early retirement, they had considerably more time to spend together than they had throughout their married life. This caused significant tension because Ms. B found her husband to be rigid. They argued frequently about small matters. Their three children had all moved away from home, and she felt as though her life was empty without her role as a parent. She had never consulted a psychiatrist but recalled that her sister had experienced several episodes of major depression, which had responded to a tricyclic antidepressant.

Ms. B's physician prescribed an antidepressant (nortriptyline 100 mg/day), which resulted in gradual improvement in her mood and anxiety. However, her sleep, concentration, and memory remained poor. Her menstrual periods had been infrequent and irregular during the past year, and she had had several hot flashes. Her physician prescribed an estrogen-progesterone oral preparation; Ms. B reported improvement in her sleep and cognitive symptoms at a follow-up visit 1 month later.

Treatment Recommendations

The management of emotional and behavioral disturbances during menopause requires an understanding of a patient's symptoms and the hormonal milieu in which they occur, her personal and family history of psychiatric illness, her current life stressors, and her attitudes toward aging and menopause. Longitudinal daily monitoring of psychic and somatic symptoms provides valuable information about the severity, stability, and pattern of symptom experience. (Many perimenopausal women experience more symptoms shortly before their menstrual period would have occurred.) Measurements of estradiol and luteinizing and follicle-stimulating hormones document the presence of menopause and hypoestrogenism. An empathic interview elicits thoughts and feelings about the subjective experience of menopause.

If a patient presents with mild depressive, anxiety, or cognitive symptoms, as well as somatic symptoms of estrogen deficiency (e.g., vaginal dryness, hot flashes), hormone replacement therapy may be prescribed as a first-line treatment, unless there are contraindications to estrogen use (e.g., breast cancer) (see also Chapters 6 and 7). If symptoms fluctuate diurnally, transdermal rather than oral estrogen may improve this pattern. However, if depressive symptoms are moderate to severe, and somatic symptoms are mild or minimal, antidepressant treatment instead of, or in addition to, hormone replacement may be the treatment of choice, especially if the patient has a personal or family history of affective disorders. (See also Chapter 9 on psychotherapeutic management of psychological symptoms in menopause.)

In surgically menopausal women, the symptoms of estrogen deficiency are often more marked than in naturally menopausal women because of the sudden decline in ovarian function. In the absence of contraindications, estrogen replacement may be particularly beneficial for these women. Also, the psychological effect of hysterectomy and bilateral oophorectomy and the reasons that necessitated the surgery must be explored.

Women who have preexisting psychotic illnesses have been poorly studied during menopause. Clinical experience suggests that some become more symptomatic at menopause. No scientifically sound studies of estrogen augmentation of antipsychotic medications have yet been done.

In patients who are already taking hormone replacement, the relation between the onset of psychological symptoms and hormone use should be evaluated. In some women, depressive, anxiety, and/or psychosomatic symptoms may result from inadequate estrogen replacement and may remit with adjustments in dosage or a change to another form of estrogen (e.g., estradiol versus conjugated estrogens, or transdermal patch versus oral administration) (Schmidt and Rubinow 1991). In other women, these symptoms may be a direct result of hormone use, especially when sequential hormone replacement is used, and may remit with a change to continuous combination therapy (Schmidt and Rubinow 1991). A small number of women are unable to tolerate the negative mood effects of progestin therapy and may prefer to take unopposed estrogen under careful observation (see Chapter 7).

Conclusion

Menopause does not appear to be characterized by an excess of clinically significant emotional or behavioral disorders or a specific menopause-related psychiatric syndrome. In contrast, minor depressive, anxiety, and psychosomatic symptoms seem to be more frequent in perimenopausal women seeking treatment for physical symptoms related to menopause (Stewart et al. 1992). For those women who do experience psychological distress in this context, it is unclear whether there is a causal connection between the onset of menopause and the occurrence of these symptoms. Recent research provides some support for the existence of a subgroup of women who are vulnerable to affective illness at times of normal gonadal hormonal changes. Moreover, considerable evidence indicates that estrogen has a complex influence on mood and cognition. Some psychological symptoms are relieved by estrogen replacement therapy, whereas others require psychotropic medication. Further research is needed to clarify the etiological and therapeutic roles of hormones and the most effective use of psychotropic medications and hormone augmentation in those women who have psychiatric disorders during menopause.

References

Alyward M: Plasma tryptophan levels and mental depression in postmenopausal subjects: effects of oral piperazine-estrone sulfate. IRCS Journal of Medical Science 1:30–34, 1973
Alyward M: Estrogens and plasma tryptophan levels in perimenopausal patients, in The Management of Menopause and Postmenopausal Years. Edited by Campbell S. Baltimore, MD, University Park Press, 1976, pp 135–147

American Psychiatric Association: Diagnostic and Statistical Manual of Mental Disorders, 3rd Edition. Washington, DC, American Psychiatric Association, 1980

Backstrom T: Estrogen and progesterone in relation to different activities in the central nervous system. Acta Obstet Gynecol Scand 66:1–17, 1977

Ballinger CB: Psychiatric morbidity and the menopause: screening of a general population sample. BMJ 3:344–346, 1975

Ballinger CB: Psychiatric aspects of the menopause. Br J Psychiatry 156:773–787, 1990

Bungay GT, Vessey MP, McPherson CK: Study of symptoms in middle life with special reference to the menopause. BMJ 144:28–34, 1980

Campbell S: Double-blind psychometric studies on the effects of natural estrogens on postmenopausal women, in The Management of Menopause and Postmenopausal Years. Edited by Campbell S. Baltimore, MD, University Park Press, 1976, pp 149–158

Campbell S, Whitehead M: Estrogen therapy and the menopause syndrome. Clin Obstet Gynecol 4:31–47, 1977

Cooke DJ: Psychosocial vulnerability to life events during the climacteric. Br J Psychiatry 147:71–75, 1985

Dennerstein L, Burrows GD: A review of the studies of psychological symptoms found at the menopause. Maturitas 1:55–64, 1978

Dennerstein L, Burrows GD, Hyman GJ, et al: Hormone therapy and affect. Maturitas 1:247–259, 1979

Derogatis LR, Spencer PM: Brief Symptom Inventory: Administration and Scoring Procedures Manual 1. Baltimore, MD, John Hopkins University Press, 1982

Deutsch H: Epilogue: the climacterium, in The Psychology of Women: A Psychoanalytic Interpretation, Vol 2. New York, Grune & Stratton, 1945, pp 456–487

Ditkoff EC, Crary WG, Cristo M, et al: Estrogen improves psychological function in asymptomatic postmenopausal women. Obstet Gynecol 78:991–995, 1991

Greene JG, Cooke DJ: Life stress and symptoms at the climacterium. Br J Psychiatry 136:486–491, 1980

Hällström T, Samuelsson S: Mental health in the climacteric. Acta Obstet Gynecol Scand 130:13–18, 1985

Holst J, Backstrom T, Hammerback S, et al: Progesterone addition during estrogen replacement therapy—effects on vasomotor symptoms and mood. Maturitas 11:13–20, 1989

Hunter M, Battersby R, Whitehead M: Relationships between psychological symptoms, somatic complaints and menopausal status. Maturitas 8:217–228, 1986

Jaszmann L, van Lith NS, Zatt JCA: The perimenopausal symptoms: the statistical analysis of a survey. Medical Gynecology and Sociology 4:268–277, 1969

Kaufert PA: The menopausal woman and her use of health services. Maturitas 2:191–206, 1980

Kelly MJ, Moss RL, Dudley CA, et al: The specificity of the response of preoptic-septal area neurons to estrogen: 17-β estradiol vs. 17-α estradiol and the response of extrahypothalamic neurons. Exp Brain Res 30:43–52, 1977

Kendall DA, Stancel AM, Enna SJ: Imipramine: effect of ovarian steroids on modifications in serotonin receptor binding. Science 211:1183–1185, 1981

Klaiber EL, Broverman DM, Vogel W, et al: Estrogen therapy for severe persistent depression in women. Arch Gen Psychiatry 36:550–554, 1979

Kraepelin E: Psychiatrie: ein Lehrbuch fur Studierende und Aerzte, 5 Aufl. Leipzig, A Abel, 1896

Leidy LE: Biological aspects of menopause: across the lifespan. Annual Review of Anthropology 23:231–253, 1994

Lock M: Introduction. Cult Med Psychiatry 10:1–5, 1986

Luine VN, McEwen BS: Effect of estradiol on turnover of type A monoamine oxidase in brain. J Neurochem 28:1221–1227, 1977

McEwen BS: The brain as a target organ of endocrine hormones, in Neuroendocrinology. Edited by Kreiger DT, Hughes JS. Sunderland, MA, Sinauer Association, 1980, pp 33–42

McEwen BS, Biegon A, Fischette CT, et al: Towards a neurochemical basis of steroid hormone action, in Frontiers in Neuroendocrinology. Edited by Martini L, Ganong W. New York, Raven, 1984, pp 1153–1176

McKinlay JB, McKinlay SM, Brambilla D: The relative contributions of endocrine changes and social circumstances to depression in mid-aged women. J Health Soc Behav 28:345–363, 1987

McKinlay SM, Jeffreys M: The menopausal syndrome. British Journal of Preventative Social Medicine 28:108–115, 1974

McKinlay SM, McKinlay JB: Health status and health care utilization by menopausal women, in Aging, Reproduction and the Climacteric. Edited by Mastroienin L, Paulsen CA. New York, Plenum, 1985

Montgomery JC, Appleby L, Brincat M, et al: Effect of estrogen and testosterone implants on psychological disorders in the climacteric. Lancet 1:297–299, 1987

Neugarten BL, Kraines RJ: 'Menopausal symptoms' in women of various
ages. Psychosom Med 27:266–273, 1965

O'Hara MW, Schlechte JA, Lewis DA, et al: Prospective study of postpartum blues: biological and psychosocial factors. Arch Gen Psychiatry
48:801–806, 1991

O'Malley BW, Means AR: Female steroid hormones and target cell nuclei.
Science 183:610–620, 1974

Parry BL: Reproductive-related depressions in women: phenomenon of
hormonal kindling?, in Postpartum Psychiatric Illness: A Picture Puz-
zle. Edited by Hamilton JA, Harberger PN. Philadelphia, University
of Pennsylvania Press, 1992, pp 200–218

Phillips S, Sherwin BB: Effects of estrogen on memory function in surgically menopausal women. Psychoneuroendocrinology 17:485–495,
1992

Prange AJ, Wilson IC, Breese GR, et al: Hormonal alteration of imipramine
response: a review, in Hormones, Behavior and Psychopathology. Edited by Sachar EJ. New York, Raven, 1976, pp 41–67

Schmidt PJ, Rubinow DR: Menopause-related affective disorders: a justification for further study. Am J Psychiatry 148:844–852, 1991

Schneider HPG: Estriol and the menopause: clinical results from a prospective study, in The Menopause: Clinical, Endocrinological and
Pathophysiological Aspects. Edited by Fioretti P, Martini L, Melis GB,
et al. New York, Academic Press, 1982, pp 523–533

Shapira B, Oppenheim G, Zohar J, et al: Lack of efficacy of estrogen supplementation to imipramine in resistant female depressives. Biol Psychiatry 20:576–579, 1985

Sherwin BB: Affective changes with estrogen and androgen replacement
therapy in surgically menopausal women. J Affect Disord 14:177–187,
1988a

Sherwin BB: Estrogen and/or androgen replacement therapy and cognitive functioning in surgically menopausal women. Psychoneuroendocrinology 10:325–335, 1988b

Sherwin BB: The impact of different doses of estrogen and progestin on
mood and sexual behavior in postmenopausal women. J Clin Endocrinol Metab 72:336–343, 1991

Sherwin BB: Impact of the changing hormonal milieu on psychological functioning, in Treatment of the Postmenopausal Woman: Basic and Clinical Aspects. Edited by Lobo RA. New York, Raven, 1994, pp 119–127

Sherwin BB, Gelfand MM: Sex steroids and affect in the surgical menopause: a double-blind, cross-over study. Psychoneuroendocrinology 10:325–335, 1985

Sherwin BB, Suranyi-Cadotte BE: Up-regulation of estrogen on platelet 3H-imipramine binding sites in surgically menopausal women. Biol Psychiatry 28:339–348, 1990

Stahl M: Role of hormone therapies for refractory depression. American Psychiatric Association Annual Meeting Proceedings, 1996, p 285

Steiner M: Female-specific mood disorders. Clin Obstet Gynecol 35:599–611, 1992

Stewart DE, Boydell K: Psychologic distress during menopause: associations across the reproductive life cycle. Int J Psychiatry Med 23:157–162, 1993

Stewart DE, Boydell K, Derzko C, et al: Psychologic distress during the menopausal years in women attending a menopause clinic. Int J Psychiatry Med 22:213–220, 1992

Thompson B, Hart S, Durno D: Menopausal age and symptomatology in general practice. J Biosoc Sci 5:71–82, 1973

Warner P, Bancroft J, Dixson A, et al: The relationship between perimenstrual depressive mood and depressive illness. J Affect Disord 23:9–23, 1991

Weisbader H, Kurzrok R: The menopause: a consideration of the symptoms, etiology and treatment by means of estrogen. Endocrinology 23:32–38, 1983

Weissman MM: The myth of involutional melancholia. JAMA 242:742–744, 1979

Winokur G: Depression in the menopause. Am J Psychiatry 130:92–93, 1973

CHAPTER 9

Psychological Treatments

Nada L. Stotland, M.D.

*M*enopause, in and of itself, is not a disease and does not require psychological treatment(s). Psychiatric illness can and does occur at every stage of life, and its preoccupations and effects are shaped by current life events. This is true for menopause as well. Menopause is an episode of hormonal and physical changes, which have considerable psychological meaning, at least for some people and cultures (see Gise, Chapter 3, and Weber, Chapter 4, in this volume). Other changes in women's lives often occur at approximately the same time as menopause: the advent of middle age, the maturation of children and their departure from home (or failure to leave when leaving is expected), the aging and infirmity of parents and other relatives, changes in employment status, and changes in intimate relationships (Barnett 1984). One change lies at the intersection of biological and social factors: the end of reproductive capacity. (Charney and Stewart focus on psychiatric aspects in Chapter 8, Robinson and Stirtzinger deal with psychoeducational and support groups for menopausal women in Chapter 10, and Jensvold reviews psychopharmacology in Chapter 11 of this volume.) In this chapter, I elaborate the issues of particular importance to the psychotherapist working with a woman of menopausal age or status and conclude with brief descriptions of the genres of psychotherapy used with this population of patients.

The social construction and implications of menopause are largely culture bound, with vast differences between cultures (see Chapter 4). In some Asian societies, women achieve positions of respect in their families only as mothers of adult sons and grand-mothers of their sons' children. They may have considerable power over daughters-in-law, who live with and serve them, and considerable influence over family decisions. Reverence for age and wisdom is a tradition.

In Western tradition, in contrast, aging women are demonized as witches or dismissed as "little old ladies." They dye their white hair brown or blond or blue, undergo surgical procedures to remove signs of maturity, risk losing their jobs, and take pains to maintain a youthful zest and facility for sexual activity lest their lovers seek new partners. This denigration of natural aging, this refusal to accept the inevitable, cannot help but have an effect on their emotional experience (Miller 1994) (see also Gise, Chapter 3, and Feldman and Netz, Chapter 12, in this volume).

Menopause, and the associated maturation, can also be liberating. Freed from the pressures of fulfilling stereotypes of female beauty and submissiveness, sometimes for the first time in their lives, women can revel in their strengths and in the discovery of new talents. Secure in both their personhood and their femininity, they may assert themselves in the workplace and the family without fear or concern of being considered masculine and overbearing (Nadelson et al. 1982). The departure of children can provide time for the deepening of friendships, interests, and intimate relationships.

Social and Historical Context

The experience of the perimenopause is largely dependent on the social context in which it occurs (see Chapters 3 and 4). Human beings are inherently social beings, with an investment in satisfying the role expectations of their cultures and subcultures (Sherwin 1993). Women in most societies are especially sensitive to the needs and expectations of their families and social institutions. Cultural and social beliefs about menopausal or aging women will be reified in the signs, symptoms, and behaviors of individual women and families.

It is virtually impossible to separate the meanings and experience of menopause from those of the aging process (see Chapter

12). Social attitudes about and roles of older women vary greatly among cultures and subcultures (Anthony 1980). In addition, there is a gender differential. The man in his 50s, 60s, and 70s, particularly if he has wealth or power, still commands not only respect but also sexual appeal. He may consort with younger women and/or men; in fact, access to beautiful young people may be seen as one of the prerogatives of his position. Women who have younger lovers tend to be ostracized. The witch, who is a hideous elderly woman often wreaking vengeance on the still fertile and attractive, is a common figure in folklore and myth.

In past generations, older women were important as bearers of knowledge about parturition and infant care and as part of the community of women who participated in child care and domestic duties. Like athletes and dancers, women who were no longer able to bear children became teachers, coaches, and supporters of those who followed. Recently, birthing and child care practices have changed so quickly that the experiences and advice of the older generation seem to the younger not only irrelevant but also dangerously outdated. Generations may clash over birthing and parenting practices, and grandmothers are relegated to observation and help with domestic chores.

Immediate Context

Against the background of the general social and historical context, the woman during perimenopause lives in the context of her own family, work, religion, and friends. These factors may or may not comport with one another and with her own feelings and preferences. The psychotherapist must be or become familiar with the context and its effects on the patient. Who has decided that the patient needs psychotherapy: her children, her primary physician, her husband or lover, her mother, or herself (Phillips 1990)? Why did this person decide that the patient needed psychotherapy? Does she or someone important to her expect menopause to cause psychiatric derangement? Menopause is frequently so depicted in the entertainment and news media and in the folklore of Western society.

The following questions must be explored: How has the loss of fertility and the maturation process affected the regard and respect she receives and expects to receive? How does she feel about menopause itself and about other aspects of the stage of life and circumstances in which she now finds herself? Does her current experience fulfill her prior expectations, positive or negative? Has she been told by her physician that menopause is a "deficiency disease" that will cause uncomfortable symptoms and bodily deterioration? How does she feel about hormonal treatment, and do her preferences match those of her primary care provider? (See Mogul, Chapter 6, and Shapiro, Chapter 7, in this volume.)

Rapid social changes and mixing of various cultural subgroups often produce discordant environments for an individual patient. For example, a woman may look forward to freedom from family responsibilities and increased opportunities for other talents and interests when she reaches menopausal age, whereas her husband may resent her outside interests, and her children may expect her to be available on demand to care for their children. Another woman may look forward to retirement from the paid workforce, whereas her significant others may object to her "vegetating" at home. Because some women were expected to subordinate their own educational and vocational preparations to those of others in their families, they may find themselves ineligible for the exciting life changes other women are boasting of. Husbands who retire intrude on their wives' autonomy and privacy at home during the hours they used to be at work. The psychotherapist must acknowledge the effects of context, help the patient to examine her assumptions, and not inadvertently reinforce negative expectations of menopause.

Case 1

Ms. U was a 55-year-old woman whose husband insisted she seek professional help because she was irritable and exhausted. He was certain these symptoms were the result of "the change." His mother had been psychiatrically hospitalized in middle age. The history obtained by the psychotherapist revealed that the patient was experiencing hot flushes, which occasionally awakened her during the night. However, she was also working part-time, performing all the domestic responsibilities in her large house, and caring for two young grandchildren 20 hours a week while her daughter went to college. The onset of her symptoms coincided with the beginning of the college term.

Psychodynamics of the Particular Patient

Each woman approaches menopause with her own history, character style, and unresolved conflicts. Because menopause embodies the end of the capacity to conceive and bear children, this phase reawakens the dynamics of the woman's relationship with her own mother. The end of a life phase invites reflection on its fulfillments and disappointments. The childhood comparison and rivalry with mother have now reached a triumphant, acceptant, or defeated conclusion. The patient may have promised herself to have more or fewer offspring than her mother or to have no children at all. Childbearing may have been perceived as the expression of her mother's enslavement or her mother's life-giving omnipotence. How has the patient's mothering compared with that of her own mother and with the mothering she fantasized before embarking on her reproductive career? Menstruation may have signified a healthy and powerful fertility or a demeaning, uncomfortable uncleanliness and deficiency. Dynamics, of course, are not mutually exclusive; opposites coexist in the unconscious.

Another aspect of oedipal rivalry is the rivalry for a loving sexual partner. This aspect of menopause stimulates dynamics of healthy and pathological narcissism. Does the woman feel secure enough in her value as a human being to transcend fears of abandonment when her youthful appearance and functions change? Her identification with her mother's aging—whether contented, bitter, or desolate—consciously and unconsciously affects her experience of menopause. Menopause can represent a punishment for her youthful triumph over her own menopausal mother.

Both individual psychology and circumstances determine the implications of the psychophysiological manifestations of menopause. Flushing red and perspiring in the middle of a board meeting, family gathering, or social event reveal otherwise intimate physical changes to everyone present. Fanning oneself or opening a window calls further attention to the situation; not doing so leads to further physical discomfort. Control and appearance are especially important to some people. Visible, uncontrollable bodily functions are humiliating. A woman whose sleep is interrupted by menopausal symptoms is in an analogous psychosocial bind. She can either take pains to hide the resulting sleepiness and irritability, make up an excuse, or tell the truth—and risk reinforcing negative social constructions of menopause and concerns about her level of functioning.

Menopause, as the end of a youthful physiological function, also signifies aging and impending death, raising existential dynamic issues for every woman. Has she been a "good" or "bad" person? What has her life meant? What do the coming years hold? Again, her own mother's experience looms large in her expectations. There is also the question of her treatment of her own mother as she aged. Will her children be devoted, disgusted, or absent? If she has no children, will menopause reawaken agonizing disappointment over infertility, or will others' accusations of "selfishness" be realized in a lonely old age?

It is as yet unclear how the advent of new reproductive treatments and technologies will affect the dynamics of menopause. News reports of postmenopausal women bearing children by hormonal stimulation and ovum donation have reached much of the Western world. Women have borne children who are genetically their daughters', when their daughters were physically incapable of doing so, in order to provide their daughters with children and themselves with grandchildren. Postmenopausal women have also chosen to bear children in new relationships or after the loss of grown children. Scientific developments disrupt the physical and emotional concept of menopause itself.

Categories of Psychological Treatment

Most readers will be familiar with the forms of treatment described and discussed below. Some basics are offered for the primary care provider or subspecialist with less exposure to the range of modalities.

Psychoanalysis

Psychoanalysis is an intense psychological treatment that aims to uncover unconscious conflicts through the exploration of the relationship with the analyst to allow the individual to make more independent, mature, and satisfying choices and relationships. The patient endeavors to say anything that comes to mind. Her train of associations is found to lead inexorably to the repressed thoughts and feelings that are the root of her symptoms. The therapist attempts to impose as little direction as possible but rather helps the patient to discern patterns and meanings in her own spontaneous thoughts (Glover 1955).

The menopausal woman brings particular concerns to psychoanalysis and psychoanalytic psychotherapy. The nondirective approach of psychoanalysis can be disconcerting to women long accustomed to more authoritarian styles in their health care providers. Older women may not be aware of the evolution of psychoanalytic theory and practice and may therefore expect what they imagine to be a strictly Freudian style and interpretation. On the other hand, maturity may enhance a woman's appreciation for the freedom of psychoanalysis.

There are several schools of psychoanalysis; the following holds for all or most of them. In general, the treatment requires three to four sessions a week for 4 years or more. Psychoanalysis is practiced by psychiatrists, psychologists, social workers, and, sometimes, lay practitioners. Psychoanalysts are not always officially licensed as such but receive credentials from their training institutes and professional associations.

Psychoanalysis is indicated when a patient has persistent and pervasive symptoms that cause pain and interfere with her ability to form mutually satisfying relationships and/or seek gratifying career or recreational pursuits. The indications for psychoanalysis do not fall into specific diagnostic categories; often, they would be diagnosed as dysphorias, personality disorders, or anxiety disorders. The patient must have considerable motivation, scheduling flexibility, and organizational capacity to maintain intensive treatment over time. She must be deeply interested in her own psychic functioning.

Psychoanalysis was once believed to be not suitable for middle-age or older persons, because their characters were too entrenched, but psychoanalysis has been used successfully with persons of all ages. A menopausal woman may not want to make this kind of investment of time, may be reluctant to examine comfortable character patterns, or may relish the prospect of focusing on self-understanding after many years of experience and frustration. Psychoanalysis at this stage of life can be a rich gift to oneself, offering the possibility to concentrate on one's own needs, feelings, and capacities after a lifetime of addressing those of others. Psychoanalytic treatment is available on an ability-to-pay basis from some of the training institutes in large metropolitan areas.

Case 2

Ms. B, a 50-year-old executive, was financially successful, was widely admired, and had a wide circle of friends, but she felt empty, as though her outward success was a sham. She complained that she was unable to enjoy the compliments showered on her. She always felt the need to accomplish greater and greater things to continue the flow of admiration, because she could not accord herself any respect. She did not feel comfortable sharing her real feelings with her social circle; the relationships were superficial. She eagerly embraced the recommendation of psychoanalysis, stating that "it is time to do something for my inner self after all these years of pursuing outward success."

In the course of the analysis, Ms. B recognized that she had always felt that her parents insisted she perform rather than concerning themselves with her needs and feelings. She reawakened interests that her parents had discouraged many years before. As she pursued those interests, she met people who valued her for them rather than for her financial and social success. Her mood improved, her anxiety decreased, and her migraine headaches diminished.

Psychodynamic Psychotherapy

Psychodynamic psychotherapy is based on the principles of psychoanalysis: the uncovering of unconscious conflicts that are remnants of past experiences and that exert an irrational, disabling influence on ongoing function. Psychodynamic psychotherapy, like psychoanalysis, requires a curious and somewhat insightful patient, but its schedule and aims are more limited than psychoanalysis. Sessions occur once or twice a week; more distant spacing can sometimes be accommodated but tends to attenuate the necessary concentration on the psychotherapeutic work. Psychodynamic psychotherapy is suitable for situations in which the patient is less disabled or motivated than the candidate for psychoanalysis or in which psychoanalysis is not practicable.

Psychodynamic psychotherapy can be lengthy or brief, open-ended or time-limited. The choice among these alternatives is determined by the training, experience, and preferences of the practitioner; the wishes and resources of the patient; and the clinical problem itself. Generally, the length of treatment required is directly proportional to the length of time the symptom has persisted. As symptoms persist, the individual and her significant others modify their activities and relationships to address or avoid them, adding secondary and tertiary problems to the original one. Treatment begun long after onset of the symptoms must address these accretions as well as the original symptom.

There is little empirical evidence for greater efficacy of longer-term psychotherapy in comparison with more limited versions (Docherty 1989). This lack of evidence does not prove that more intensive and longer therapies are not more useful; longer treatments are more difficult to study than shorter treatments, because the problems treated are more complex, and there are many more intervening variables, such as the effect of environmental forces on the patient's recovery. During the course of several years, relatives are born and die, jobs are gained and lost, and friends move closer or farther away. As the patient's condition improves, the changes in her mood and behavior alter the responses she receives from the environment.

Open-ended psychodynamic psychotherapy has much in common with psychoanalysis; the therapist tends not to direct the focus of treatment but to allow the flow of the patient's thoughts to enlighten them both about her inner dynamics, the sources of her difficulties, and her personal choices for the future. Similarly, the menopausal woman suitable for open-ended treatment will have considerable interest in her own psyche, the capacity to tolerate ambiguity, resources of time and money, and patience. Open-ended psychodynamic psychotherapy is suitable for the treatment of long-standing problems with interpersonal relationships, career goals, and self-esteem. A menopausal woman may enter a psychotherapy relationship at the time of a crisis, such as a divorce, and, intrigued by the possibility of knowing herself better and resolving lifelong problems, will continue the treatment after the immediate crisis has passed.

Some psychodynamic psychotherapists believe that all such treatment should be rigorously focused on a narrowly defined symptom or problem (Levenson and Butler 1994). These psychotherapists use psychodynamic understanding but are much more directive than the psychoanalyst (MacKenzie 1991). A goal and number of sessions—generally 6–12—for treatment are agreed on by patient and therapist at the outset (Binder et al. 1987). Time-limited therapies are suitable for acute and defined problems, such as new-onset depression, anxiety, and somatic symptoms.

Case 3

Ms. C, a 45-year-old woman, had worked at the same clerical job for 15 years. When her company underwent a reorganization, it became apparent that she had acquired, over the years, experience, knowledge, and skills that were critical to its future success. She was promoted into a management position, with a salary exceeding that of her husband and the members of her family of origin. Her children were proud and supportive. Her own response, however, seemed paradoxical; she felt insecure, anxious, and depressed. Her husband attributed her symptoms to "the change of life." In the course of psychotherapy, she realized that she harbored an unconscious conviction that her success could only be achieved at significant cost to her loved ones. She was then able to manage both her competitive feelings and theirs. Her symptoms abated, and she enjoyed her new role.

Supportive Psychotherapy

Supportive psychotherapy is indicated for the patient who is not interested, capable, and/or in need of discovering why she is upset or dysfunctional. Little or no attempt is made to make her consciously aware of her underlying conflicts. The foregoing statement does not imply that an understanding of those conflicts, and the defensive mechanisms the patient uses to contain them, is not useful, or even essential, to the therapist. Supportive psychotherapy is suitable for acute or chronic crisis, such as situations in which external circumstances or personal illness threatens to overwhelm the patient's functioning either temporarily or permanently. The therapist determines what external and internal resources the patient brings to the situation and helps her to mobilize and utilize them (Ursano and Silberman 1994). Supportive psychotherapy can be extremely valuable to the menopausal patient beset by external problems: an unsupportive work or family environment, a loss, and the need to care for dependent family members.

Case 4

Ms. D's lesbian lover of 20 years died suddenly when Ms. D was age 52. Her lover had managed the business affairs of the household. Ms. D was not only bereaved and lonely but also terrified at the prospect of maintaining her house, deciding among insurance policies, and providing for her retirement. She was frequently tearful and appeared distraught. Her therapist helped her to seek advice from knowledgeable friends, to take one task at a time, to call on her willing family to provide emotional support and company, and to put her responsibilities in perspective, recognizing that her grief had colored her ability to manage them with her more-than-adequate intellect.

Interpersonal Therapy

Interpersonal therapy is based on the premise that human beings are intensely social creatures, whose development, self-esteem, and contentment are closely related to their relationships with others. The interpersonal therapist concentrates on the social aspects of the patient's history, current life situation, symptoms, and dysfunction. Because interpersonal therapy was developed as a treatment of mild or moderate cases of depression, the therapist also will inquire about common concomitants of that disorder, including changing life roles, interpersonal disagreements, social deficits, and bereavement. Therapy focuses on discordance between the patient's and others' perceptions of her behavior, on the difficulties caused by the patient's negative expectations of social situations, on the clarification of the patient's interpersonal wishes and needs, and on the improvement of interpersonal communication (Marmar et al. 1989).

Behavior Therapies

Behavior therapies were based on observations that behavior could be modified by altering the context in which a person functioned. Behaviorists questioned the necessity or efficacy of the attempt to understand the unconscious origins and motivations of a person's dysfunction when a simple change in behavior could relieve the problem. They noted that emotions, physiological responses, and behaviors become associated with environmental cues, which are related in time but not in substance.

Patients may develop anger, sadness, phobias, avoidance, anxiety, and other symptoms in response to environmental cues that were coincidentally present during an experience in which those reactions were normative. For example, a patient undergoing nausea-producing chemotherapy for a malignancy will often develop nausea at the mere sight or smell of the treatment center or even on the way there. A patient's blood pressure may rise whenever she smells aftershave lotion that reminds her of an abusive ex-husband. Behavioral interventions are aimed at breaking the association, often by substituting a neutral or more positive one; for example, the smell of aftershave can be associated with going out, meeting people, and enjoying oneself. Repeated, graduated exposure to an aversive stimulus can extinguish the behavioral response; for example, the patient who is afraid of elevators practices getting in and out of an elevator with the door open, then opening and closing the door, then riding up or down one floor with a trusted companion, and so forth.

Behaviors are also affected by the responses they evoke. A laboratory rat may press a pedal because pellets of food are released, a toddler may whine because he is given otherwise forbidden candy when he whines, and an adult patient who dislikes or resents certain errands may lose her car keys so that she is relieved of those errands by other people. These responses are automatic, not deliberate or consciously manipulative. The behavior is said to be reinforced by the environmental response that leads to its repetition. Secondarily, the patient may elicit attention, concern, companionship, or other reinforcers as a result of her symptoms or dysfunction. The behavior therapist helps the patient and her significant others to analyze the circumstances in which the problematic behavior occurs and to reconstruct the circumstances so that they no longer reinforce the behavior (Agras and Berkowitz 1994; O'Leary and Wilson 1987). For example, the patient may decide she will have to take the bus to complete her errands if her car keys are missing. Family members will not comment or help her search for them. They will show interest and pleasure when she develops a plan to keep track of the keys successfully.

Cognitive Therapy

Cognitive therapy is behavior therapy that focuses on the patient's thought content and thought processes rather than on overt behaviors. Cognitive therapy is based on the observation that much psychological suffering and dysfunction are associated with historically derived, but currently counterproductive, thought patterns. The following joke illustrates this paradigm:

> A person's car develops a flat tire on a trip to the country. He does not have the jack needed to replace the tire, so he sets off for a nearby farmhouse to ask if he can borrow one. As he walks, he imagines the negative response he may receive when he knocks at the door. By the time he reaches the house, he has convinced himself that his request will be denied and has worked himself into a rage at the prospect. The farmer, who would have been perfectly willing to lend his jack and assist the motorist, is met at his front door with a fuming man who shouts, "Keep your *!#/ jack! I don't want it anyway."

An individual who is depressed anticipates negative responses and blames her misery on her own failings: "I don't deserve a raise," "No one will like me," "Nothing good will ever happen to me." Such erroneous thoughts lead to behaviors that, indeed, provoke the anticipated negative outcomes (Casey and Grant 1992). She does not share her good ideas at work, invite her friends over, or plan activities she would enjoy. In cognitive therapy, she learns to identify her counterproductive and incorrect thoughts and their negative outcomes. She practices recognizing those cognitions whenever they occur and actively substituting more accurate and optimistic thoughts each time. Improving her thoughts benefits her behaviors and her moods (Wright and Beck 1994). Cognitive therapy, like other behavior therapies, is highly structured, time limited, and goal oriented.

Couples Therapy

Couples therapy can be utilized with married or unmarried and same- or opposite-sex couples. It is used when a patient's complaints or symptoms focus on her interactions with her partner. Couples therapy can be informed by psychodynamic understanding, but its focus is behavioral. The therapist helps the two participants to deflect their energy from complaints and arguments to affirming each other's positive attributes, practicing more effective communication, and making mutual agreements to change the behaviors that perturb each other.

Family Therapy

Many family therapists believe that most or all dysfunction arises from the matrix of the family. The person with the symptoms merely expresses, or is the scapegoat for, the dysfunction of the family. For example, a menopausal woman may become depressed, and be identified as mentally ill, because of unresolved, unremitting conflict between her husband and one of their children. Family therapy includes as many generations and individuals as possible. The therapist is able to observe family interactions as they occur and to offer interpretations, insights, and suggestions not only or especially to the designated "patient," but also to whomever is appropriate or to the family in general. As in couples therapy, which is a variant of family therapy, the family may be given "homework," which involves practicing new ways of communicating, listening, and behaving (Rolland and Walsh 1994).

Group Therapies

For a discussion of group therapies, please refer to Chapter 10 in this volume.

Matching the Treatment to the Patient

Few clinical situations offer the complete range of psychotherapeutic treatments described above. Too often, the type of psychotherapy a patient receives is dictated by the clinical philosophy and experience of the particular setting where she happens to seek treatment and by financial and reimbursement issues rather than by her needs and preferences. It is preferable to determine which types of psychotherapy would meet the patient's needs and secondarily to consider the realities of what is available.

The length of time since onset of the symptoms is grossly correlated with the probable length of time required to resolve the symptoms. The patient may or may not be interested in and talented at increasing her understanding of herself, her unconscious conflicts, and the effect of her early experiences. It should not be assumed that these interests and talents are limited to the upper socioeconomic classes or to specific ethnic groups.

Some patients prefer a structured, goal-oriented therapy. Group therapies are particularly useful for patients who are facing a life problem or transition, such as menopause, that is shared by others and for those who have deficits in their social skills (see Chapter 10). Couples or family therapy is indicated for patients whose problems are focused on those relationships. Many third-party payers severely limit the indications, type of treatment, type of provider, and number of sessions for psychotherapy. The referring physician and/or psychotherapist must be specific about the indications for treatment and the treatment goals and duration.

Selection of the Therapist

In the past, a great deal of attention was paid to the selection of a therapist particularly suited to address problem areas in a patient's life; for example, an older man for a patient without a father. No real evidence indicates that this kind of selection is necessary or helpful. If a patient has a particular preference for the age, sex, sexual orientation, ethnicity, or style of therapist, the request should be honored if possible, and then the reasons for the request should be explored in the therapy itself. An insistence on a female therapist may be a sign of an exploitative relationship with a male therapist or other authority figure in the past. Patients who are pleased with their therapists tend to achieve more therapeutic benefit. Primary care physicians who are interested and trained can perform brief psychotherapy very effectively with some of their patients. Treatment by a psychiatrist is critical in cases in which there are unexplained somatic symptoms, medical and psychological diagnostic questions, and/or a need to consider or prescribe psychoactive medications concomitantly with the psychotherapy.

Initiation of Treatment

The need for outside help with psychological symptoms is experienced as a blow to self-esteem (Basch 1980). If the referral comes from a primary physician, then the physician should be careful to make the reason for the referral clear and to indicate ongoing interest in the patient by word and deed. The patient may otherwise assume that the primary physician thinks she is "crazy," is troublesome, or has physical symptoms that are "all in her head." Some patients have particularly strong prejudices and feelings about psychiatrists as compared with other psychotherapists. Going to a counselor or therapist seems to imply less severe psychopathology than going to a psychiatrist. When the clinical situation dictates the choice of a medically and psychologically trained psychotherapist, the referring professional may have to explain the reasons carefully. Most patients are reassured by an explanation that the psychiatrist has had medical training, so as to understand the physiology of menopause, the effects and side effects of medications, and the diagnosis and treatment of general medical disorders. The patient should be given an appointment to see or call the primary physician soon after the appointment with the therapist to inform the primary physician about her experience and the therapist's recommendations.

Special Circumstances

Influential, wealthy, and/or famous patients may elicit special consideration from therapists. It is reasonable to take particular care to protect their privacy, not because they deserve more privacy, but because their privacy is more likely to be invaded by curious individuals, groups, and/or media. The therapist also must take care either not to take advantage of the patient's power or to be taken advantage of; it is especially important with these patients to observe the same practice style that is used with other patients (e.g., no home visits, no special hours), except as may be absolutely necessary to protect privacy or accommodate other overwhelming demands on a patient's time.

Indigent women, on the other hand, may have no access to therapy at all. Women are at increased risk for poverty, for having no health care coverage, and for having obligations, schedules, and chaotic demands that take precedence over nonemergency health care appointments. Ethnic and minority group women may have difficulty finding a therapist who speaks their language (if they do not speak English fluently) and is knowledgeable about the psychological ramifications of menopause in their culture (see Chapter 4). This difficulty can be addressed with open communication and, if necessary, consultation with an expert. Lesbian women may seek care from lesbian therapists because they fear that "straight" therapists will make unwarranted assumptions about their lives and their psychodynamics.

Patients who express suicidal ideation at presentation should optimally be evaluated immediately by a psychiatrist. Chronic, mild suicidal ideation, without specific intent or behavior, can be handled in psychotherapy by other mental health professionals as well. Patients with disorders for which psychotropic medication is indicated (see Chapters 8–11) generally benefit substantially from psychotherapy as well. Ideally, the two forms of therapy should be provided by the same professional. At the very least, the psychotherapist should be in close, regular contact with the prescriber of medication.

A final caveat is that the intimacy and dependency of psychotherapy increase the vulnerability of patients and therapists to breach professional boundaries. It is natural for psychotherapy to provoke friendly, sexual, and many other feelings. The therapist must use these feelings as indicators of what is happening in the therapy. Any indication that the feelings may be acted on, however, is an indication for immediate consultation with an expert and possible referral of the patient to another therapist. Professional and close social/sexual relationships cannot coexist in psychotherapy; the patient ends up with neither (Bruch 1974).

References

Agras WS, Berkowitz RI: Behavior therapy, in The American Psychiatric Press Textbook of Psychiatry, 2nd Edition. Edited by Hales RE, Yudofsky SC, Talbott JA. Washington, DC, American Psychiatric Press, 1994, pp 1061–1082

Anthony EJ: Psychoanalysis and environment, in The Course of Life: Psychoanalytic Contributions Toward Understanding Personality Development, Vol III. Edited by Pollock G. Washington, DC, National Institute of Mental Health, 1980, pp 201–240

Barnett RC: The anxiety of the unknown—choice, risk, responsibility: therapeutic issues for today's adult women, in Women in Midlife. Edited by Baruch G, Brooks-Gunn J. New York, Plenum, 1984, pp 341–358

Basch MF: Doing Psychotherapy. New York, Basic Books, 1980

Binder JL, Henry WP, Strupp HH: An appraisal of selection criteria for dynamic psychotherapies and implications for setting time limits. Psychiatry 50:154–166, 1987

Bruch H: Learning Psychotherapy: Rationale and Ground Rules. Cambridge, MA, Harvard University Press, 1974

Casey DA, Grant RW: Cognitive therapy with depressed elderly inpatients, in Cognitive Therapy With Inpatients: Developing a Cognitive Milieu. Edited by Wright JH, Thase ME, Beck AT, et al. New York, Guilford, 1992, pp 295–314

Docherty JP: The individual psychotherapies: efficacy, syndrome-based treatments, and the therapeutic alliance, in Outpatient Psychiatry: Diagnosis and Treatment, 2nd Edition. Edited by Griffin LA. Baltimore, MD, Williams & Wilkins, 1989, pp 624–644

Glover E: The Technique of Psycho-Analysis. New York, International Universities Press, 1955

Levenson H, Butler SF: Brief dynamic individual psychotherapy, in The American Psychiatric Press Textbook of Psychiatry, 2nd Edition. Edited by Hales RE, Yudofsky SC, Talbott JA. Washington, DC, American Psychiatric Press, 1994, pp 1009–1033

MacKenzie KR: Principles of brief intensive psychotherapy. Psychiatric Annals 21:398–404, 1991

Marmar CR, Gaston L, Gallagher D, et al: Alliance and outcome in late-life depression. J Nerv Ment Dis 177:464–472, 1989

Miller JB: Women's psychological development: connections, disconnections, and violations, in Women Beyond Freud: New Concepts of Feminine Psychology. Edited by Berger MM. New York, Brunner/ Mazel, 1994, pp 79–98

Nadelson CC, Polonsky DC, Mathews MA: Marriage and midlife: the impact of social change, in The Woman Patient, Vol 2. Edited by Nadelson CC, Notman MT. New York, Plenum, 1982, pp 145–158

O'Leary KD, Wilson GT: Behavior Therapy: Application and Outcome, 2nd Edition. Englewood Cliffs, NJ, Prentice-Hall, 1987

Phillips SB: Reflections of self and other: men's views of menopausal women, in The Meanings of Menopause: Historical, Medical, and Clinical Perspectives. Edited by Formanek R. Hillsdale, NJ, Analytic Press, 1990, pp 281–296

Rolland JS, Walsh F: Family therapy: systems approaches to assessment and treatment, in The American Psychiatric Press Textbook of Psychiatry, 2nd Edition. Edited by Hales RE, Yudofsky SC, Talbott JA. Washington, DC, American Psychiatric Press, 1994, pp 1177–1208

Sherwin BB: Menopause: myths and realities, in Psychological Aspects of Women's Health Care. Edited by Stewart DE, Stotland NL. Washington, DC, American Psychiatric Press, 1993, pp 227–248

Ursano RJ, Silberman EK: Psychoanalysis, psychoanalytic psychotherapy, and supportive psychotherapy, in The American Psychiatric Press Textbook of Psychiatry, 2nd Edition. Edited by Hales RE, Yudofsky SC, Talbott JA. Washington, DC, American Psychiatric Press, 1994, pp 1035–1060

Wright JH, Beck AT: Cognitive therapy, in The American Psychiatric Press Textbook of Psychiatry, 2nd Edition. Edited by Hales RE, Yudofsky SC, Talbott JA. Washington, DC, American Psychiatric Press, 1994, pp 1083–1114

CHAPTER 10

Psychoeducational Programs and Support Groups at Transition to Menopause

Gail Erlick Robinson, M.D., F.R.C.P.C.
Ruth Stirtzinger, M.D., F.R.C.P.C.

*N*egative expectations of the menopause and the conviction that it presages a marked deterioration in mental health persist in Western culture (Ballinger 1990). Negative feelings about menopause have been found to be related to higher symptom reporting, higher rates of depression, and increased physical symptomatology (Avis and McKinley 1991). The woman who anticipates severe symptoms is at a greater psychological risk for distress than women who expect mild or no symptoms (Gath and Iles 1990). The effect of negative anticipation of menopause is borne out by the fact that postmenopausal women often express relief at the cessation of periods, whereas perimenopausal women are the least likely to report relief (Avis and McKinley 1991). Even if the higher levels of psychological distress found in perimenopausal women (Stewart et al. 1992) are related directly to hormonal changes, fears, uncertainty, and negative expectations can exaggerate their effect. If belief systems, misinformation, attitudes, and concurrent worries can influence the experience of menopause, then, by altering an individual's myths or negative expectations and/or helping her deal with her concerns about menopause, it should be possible to reduce both psychological and physiological distress during this transitional period (Bowles 1990).

Group programs have been found to be valuable, cost-effective approaches to dealing with shared life events. In the case of anticipated events such as menopause, they may also provide an opportunity for primary prevention. The group approach may take the form of educational, psychodynamic, support, or self-help therapy. Obviously, support is a factor in all approaches.

Educational Groups

In a study by La Rocco and Polit (1980), the largest percentage of women interviewed said that the worst thing about menopause was "not knowing what to expect." Eighty percent of women would like more information about the menopause before its onset (Roberts 1991). It is often very difficult for women to obtain accurate information about what menopause really entails. Berkun (1986) noted that women thought the information they had was inadequate and depended greatly on the variability of physicians' ability to communicate. Surveys in both Australia and North America (Abraham et al. 1995; Randall 1993) indicate that physicians often do not discuss the issues that concern women most. Physicians were most likely to discuss short-term physical symptoms, such as hot flashes, and less likely to discuss emotional symptoms, sexual functioning, heart disease, or osteoporosis. Although 67% said that their physicians discussed treatment for physical symptoms and mentioned hormone replacement therapy, other nonhormonal treatments, such as exercise, smoking cessation, diet, and stress reduction techniques, were recommended by fewer than 2% of physicians.

Most of the information supplied to the general population about climacteric complaints and how to avoid them is based on clinical experience associated with negative expectations (Holte and Mikkelsen 1991). Most women receive much of their information on menopause from nonphysician sources, mainly the media, magazines, books, and female friends and relatives (Abraham et al. 1995; Randall 1993; Roberts 1991). Information reported in the media may be inaccurate or distorted; the fact that most women cope well with menopause is not as sensational a story as the problems some women face. Not only a lack of information but also the determination of what is authentic make learning about menopause difficult (Cobb 1990). Women who try to read scientific literature may be confused by studies with conflicting results. Women want more than simple reassurance or biological facts. They want to know how to sort out controllable from uncontrollable physical and mental sensations (Berkun 1986).

Educational groups work on the assumption that providing accurate information about menopause and dispelling myths and false perceptions will reduce women's fears and concerns and, therefore, their negative experiences. Educational groups tend to be time-limited, structured, and led by professionals. Participants have ample opportunity to ask questions and share experiences.

Stirtzinger et al. (1992) reported on workshops consisting of three 3-hour sessions covering the physical, psychological, and psychosocial issues related to menopause and women at midlife. Each workshop had 20–30 participants, with a mixture of pre-, peri-, and postmenopausal women. The goals of the workshops were to dispel myths that menopause is the central event for midlife women that unilaterally changes their personalities and psychological characteristics; provide up-to-date, scientific information about the benefits and risks of hormone replacement therapy; and increase women's sense of mastery with regard to their health and life stage changes. The format included lectures, discussion periods, films, and books. The workshops were conducted by an obstetrician-gynecologist or family practitioner and a psychiatrist. The combination of a gynecologist or family practitioner and a psychiatrist allowed a unified approach to physical and psychosocial influences.

The gynecologist or family practitioner presented facts about the physiological process of menopause, including the effects of estrogen fluctuations, vasomotor theories regarding hot flashes and sweats, osteoporosis, and indications and contraindications for hormone replacement therapy. Physiological symptoms directly related to hormonal changes were differentiated from more general complaints related to aging. The relationships between stress, changing estrogen levels, and nighttime hot flashes, sweats, and sleep disturbance were also discussed. The clinician explained how interrupted sleep may be responsible for some common symptoms.

The psychiatrist focused on factors contributing to stress during this period, including increased personal losses and deaths, fears related to aging, and changes in roles. Information about the experience of menopause in women in other cultures helped to emphasize the importance of attitudes toward changes in status and life satisfaction in determining whether menopause is a positive or negative experience. The psychiatrist also presented information about the sociological and organic causes of depression to counteract the belief that menopause automatically leads to depression.

Discussion about the cognitive and emotional changes in this age group emphasized the role of stress in producing symptoms, such as memory loss, attention deficits, anxiety, and irritability, in some women; all of these symptoms are commonly attributed to the menopause. The phases of stress response as described by Caplan (1981) were discussed: the search for new behavior, the use of behaviors designed to decrease the uncomfortable emotional arousal from stress, and the alteration in thinking required to come to terms with the stressful event. The group environment allowed the women to explore their own sense of competence and their perception of present and future demands on them. They could discuss the stresses in their lives and coping strategies.

Network building and discussion among participants were important parts of the format. Early in the series, groups of seven or eight women worked on focus questions distributed by leaders. Group members were also invited to compose their own questions. These questions elicited discussion of issues such as the effect women believe the menopause will have on the rest of their lives, factors they believe will affect their experience of menopause, and the ways in which women feel they can gain control over their experience of menopause.

Questionnaires completed before and after the program indicated that the women felt significantly less anxious, less depressed, less irritable, and generally more hopeful about themselves after the workshop. The participants not only reported positive mood changes but also indicated that, even without starting hormone replacement therapy, they were bothered less by hot flashes and night sweats. Moreover, they felt less anxious about their sexuality and menopause and their general body functioning. The majority (96.4%) felt more confident about their health during menopause, and 83.3% felt more capable of finding appropriate health care. Comments from participants illustrated some of the benefits: "How sad that women have been made to feel embarrassed about a normal part of their life"; "The workshops gave me hope through understanding as I was getting discouraged with sweats and lack of sleep"; and "Through discussions at the workshop, I realized I was not alone and was not going crazy."

The women who completed follow-up questionnaires sent out 1 year after completing the workshop continued to be significantly less depressed, anxious, and irritable than before the program, indicating that the changes achieved by the workshop were long lasting. Such groups benefit from the inclusion of premenopausal, perimenopausal, and postmenopausal women so that those who have already gone through the process can share their knowledge, experience, and more positive attitudes. Stirtzinger et al. (1992) concluded that the menopausal educational workshop was effective in reducing stress and helping the participants feel more hopeful about their lives.

Anderson et al. (1987) established a menopause clinic consisting of group discussions with four to six women followed by personal counseling with each patient during the one-time, 4-hour clinic visit. The clinic was staffed by a medical anthropologist, a nurse, and a physician with special expertise in reproductive endocrinology who acted as a consultant. Topics explored in the group sessions conducted by a health professional included symptoms of the menopause, advantages and disadvantages of hormone replacement therapy, the importance of using progestins concomitantly with estrogens in women with intact uteri, cardiovascular disease, osteoporosis, surgical menopause, nutrition, exercise, breast self-examination, and mammography. Patients were encouraged to discuss their problems, fears, and frustrations. Patients received an annotated bibliography of references related to the menopause and similar topics, a diary in which to keep relevant information on the menopause, dietary and exercise information, and a monthly record sheet on which to record symptoms related to the menopause.

In the individual counseling sessions with the clinic staff, patients could discuss and receive guidance on whether to discuss hormone replacement therapy with their physician and/or seek individual consultation from a psychiatrist, a career counselor, or a nutritionist.

This approach appears to be helpful in relieving both physical and emotional symptoms (Anderson et al. 1987). Six months after clinic attendance, follow-up questionnaires were mailed to the first 100 participants and their partners, if applicable, to assess the benefits of the menopause clinic visit, actions taken subsequently, and adjustments with their partner. Most of the women attending the clinic were currently married, had children, and had some education after high school; about half were employed. More than 50% of the women reported that the reason for their appointment was primarily education and support, and 80% of the patients believed that their visit had been useful. Of those who had reported hot flashes, one-third stated that their symptoms had become less frequent and/or less intense in the interim, in most cases as a result of the use of estrogen replacement. Women stated that they had benefited from being encouraged to seek medical care, finding relief in the knowledge that many women had similar complaints and gaining helpful information about the menopause.

A second follow-up survey was sent to the 400 women who attended the menopause clinic during the years 1984–1989 (Hamburger and Anderson 1990). Of the 134 individuals who responded, 55% believed they were better able to use the services of their gynecologist, 25% their general practitioner, and 16% their internist. Only 8% mentioned seeing a psychiatrist or psychologist. When asked what changes in their lifestyle they had made since attending the clinic, 64% stated that they were using mammography at appropriate intervals, 58% reported that they were eating a low-fat/calcium-rich diet, 49% stated that they had incorporated an exercise program, and 44% claimed that they were receiving medical checkups. Patients indicated that they had a better understanding of a variety of subjects covered in the clinic, such as hormone replacement therapy (80%), osteoporosis (60%), progesterone (44%), and regular mammography (39%). Fifty-nine percent stated that their mental health had improved, and 48% claimed improvement in their physical health. Sixty-two percent said that attending the clinic had enabled them to accept this time of life. Thirty-five percent felt that they were able to plan for the future, and 18% felt that they were more productive. The percentage of women who were taking hormone replacement therapy increased from 38% to 76%, which was thought to be the result of an increased confidence about starting this therapy after having received more information. The results of their survey validated the authors' impressions that women seemed to know very little about the menopause and had difficulties separating myths from fact. The authors concluded that the clinic responded to the patients' needs for educational and emotional support, resulting in better use of the services of health professionals and lifestyle and preventive changes.

Weiss (1994) illustrated how educational/support groups can be modified to serve different populations. Her basic model was a series of educational/support programs for menopause sponsored by the Employee Wellness Program at the Mount Sinai Medical Center in New York City. Each program ran for 8 consecutive weeks at the lunch hour. Teams of interdisciplinary health care professionals addressed issues such as the medical aspects of the menopausal and the perimenopausal years, current therapeutic approaches, nutrition, exercise, sexuality, and stress management. The organizers then established a community-based program in East Harlem. This area of New York City is characterized by poverty, high unemployment, crime, poor education, and single-parent households, mainly headed by women. The stated purpose of the program was to reach desperately poor women living on the edges of society, frequently isolated from health care systems and lacking the motivation or habit of seeking information, much less making lifestyle changes compatible with good health. The organizers appreciated that these women viewed menopause as a "white middle-class problem" and that low-income minority women probably would not attend a program solely focused on menopause. The aim was to adapt the Mount Sinai program to suit this new cultural context.

A nine-session program lasting 4 months was held in the community drop-in center. A respected member of the community served as the liaison between the local women and the hospital. The program included teaching the women about stress management, female reproductive life, menopausal changes and hormone replacement therapy, gynecological and breast health, nutrition, exercise, midlife sexuality, and gaining access to helping systems. Child care and refreshments were provided. Weiss concluded that the program worked because of consistent participation by staff who became familiar to the residents, mutual sharing in the recognition of the common bonds of womanhood, adaptation of the program to the needs of the community, presentation of the educational material in understandable ways, and use of a "cultural ambassador" to act as a link between the two communities.

This program is an effective model of how an educational program can be adapted to various groups and settings (Weiss 1994). It demonstrates that the menopausal and perimenopausal years provide an excellent opportunity to develop a preventive approach to health care and well-being (Weiss 1994). It also shows that it is important to bring services into a milieu (e.g., libraries, colleges, adult educational facilities, women's clubs and organizations, community centers, and cooperative extension programs) that middle-age women find comfortable and accessible and that normalizes rather than medicalizes menopause (Berkun 1986). Establishing such programs in a wide range of settings can overcome the tendency of different groups of women to avoid resources that appear to violate dearly held values or that require the assumption of an unwanted label such as psychiatric patient or one associated with poverty (such as social agencies) or radicalism (such as a feminist health collective) (Berkun 1986).

Case 1

Ms. A was a 49-year-old mother of two children, the younger of whom had just left home to attend college. For the past 5 years, Ms. A had been developing her own business, which was starting to be very successful. At a time when her life seemed busy and happy, she began to have some menopausal symptoms. Although she was troubled by the prospect of hot flashes and night sweats, she was more concerned about her belief that most women going through menopause become depressed and irritable. She was afraid that these symptoms would jeopardize her career, her marriage, and her good relationship with her children.

Ms. A attended a three-session psychoeducational program for perimenopausal women. She was relieved to find out that many of her apprehensions about menopause were based on myths and misunderstandings. The discussion and information at the workshop helped her to understand what was happening to her body and made her realize that other women were experiencing the same symptoms and fears. She obtained information about the use of hormone replacement therapy and alternative treatments for menopausal symptoms so that she was able to make an informed decision about which approach she would use. The information that she gained in the psychoeducational workshop helped change her perspective about menopause. Rather than viewing it as a time of loss, depression, irritability, and distressing negative symptoms, she saw it as a time of reassessment and reevaluation and as an opportunity to make healthy lifestyle changes. She made an appointment for a medical checkup, changed her diet, quit smoking, and started an exercise program.

Psychodynamic Groups

The psychodynamic group approach works on the assumption that some women may have particular difficulties around the menopause because of past and current intra- and interpersonal conflicts. The end of menstruation can act as a trigger that leads to the resurgence of unresolved conflicts from earlier stages of the life cycle (Lock 1991). Eligibility requirements for psychodynamic group therapy include

- Perimenopausal state
- Emotional distress
- Psychological mindedness
- Ability to express feelings
- Motivation to change
- Willingness to commit to a weekly psychotherapy process

Exclusion criteria include

- Psychosis
- Current major depressive disorders

- Suicidal or acting-out behavior, which may interfere with the ability to work in a group
- Marked incompatibility with group norms for acceptable behavior
- Tendency to assume a deviant role
- Inability to tolerate a group setting

Groups typically include 8–10 members and are led by a trained group therapist, sometimes with a co-therapist. Groups meet on a weekly basis for 1.5–2 hours over a predetermined period ranging from 2–6 months to several years. Usually, no new members are introduced to the group once it is established.

Such groups encourage exploration and understanding of the specific meanings of this shared experience for each member. Menopause, for example, may be devastating for an individual woman who, feeling unlovable, used her sexuality to attract men in order to feel worthwhile. For such a woman, menopause may not appear as a normal developmental stage but rather heralds the beginning of abandonment and loneliness. Similarly, a woman who has viewed her sense of worth as attached to her fertility may find the cessation of menses not a relief from fear of pregnancy but the end of her value as an individual. The psychodynamically oriented group would focus on understanding the early development of such feelings of low self-worth and, with the support of other group members, helping the individual to rebuild her view of herself so she is better able to accept the changes of midlife. Therapeutic mechanisms operating in this type of group therapy include the instillation of hope, universality, catharsis, and group cohesiveness and the imparting of information and interpersonal learning.

Case 2

Ms. B, a 52-year-old divorced woman, was working as a senior executive in a large firm. Despite the fact that she was an attractive, outgoing woman with a successful career, she harbored long-standing doubts and feelings of low self-esteem. Her mother, a very bright woman who had taken the traditional route of staying home and looking after four children, would minimize Ms. B's career success and, instead, focus on the fact that Ms. B had not been able to sustain a marriage and had never had children.

When Ms. B began to experience early symptoms of menopause, she started to feel anxious and sad. She worried that having hot flashes during meetings would interfere with her ability to do her work. Her appearance had always been important to her. She saw menopause as being equivalent to aging and feared that she would no longer be viewed as attractive and would never find another partner. Although she had decided 15 years previously not to have children, she began to wonder whether she had made the right choice and to view herself as an inadequate woman for never really trying to have a family. Although Ms. B was able to control her hot flashes by starting hormone replacement therapy, her concerns about aging, loss of attractiveness, loneliness, and childlessness remained.

Ms. B was seen as an excellent candidate for psychodynamically oriented group therapy. She was motivated, intelligent, psychologically minded, and articulate. Over the course of 2 years of weekly group therapy, she was able to understand more clearly how her mother's ambivalence about her own life choice had led to her denigrating Ms. B's decisions. Ms. B began to reevaluate her life choices and to feel more confident about her success and abilities. She appreciated that her appeal to others was not merely on the basis of her physical attractiveness but on the type of person that she was. Her increased self-esteem led her to be more open and less defensive in relationships. She became involved with a new man in a healthy, mature relationship. She was able to deal with some grief about never having children but concluded that she had made the right decision for her.

Support Groups

Patient support groups help women redefine their experience more positively, increase their social network, and learn from others' progress (Dennerstein 1988).

Groups Led by Professionally Trained Leaders

Groups led by professionally trained leaders focus on the shared experience of being a woman at midlife rather than on individual dynamics. Groups meet weekly, biweekly, or monthly for a fixed or variable duration. Group members usually can join the group at any time, drop in or out of the group, or continue indefinitely.

The approach of the group is generally an empathic and positive one. The expression of individual psychopathology is neither sought nor desirable, and confrontation is avoided. Although information about menopause may be shared, the emphasis is on the emotional experience of menopause. The group may function in an unstructured manner, or various themes may be proposed for particular meetings. Discussions might center around changing roles, relationships with spouses and children, concerns about caring for older parents, or fears of aging. Cognitive-behavior therapy techniques aimed at helping women change their personal perception of the events surrounding menopause may help the participants deal with the stresses in their life (Dennerstein 1988). Relaxation techniques may also be taught.

Self-Help Groups

Self-help groups have become increasingly popular sources of information and support for individuals dealing with a variety of problems. Groups such as Alcoholics Anonymous and Recovery Inc. have proved the value of such approaches. Self-help groups meet every 1–4 weeks. Groups are open-ended, and participants attend as they wish. Group leaders are individuals who have experienced the same difficulties as the other participants. Groups led by women who are not physicians and who are near, or at, the climacteric provide a positive role model, indicating that normality, strength, and vitality are natural qualities of the middle years (Berkun 1986). Leaders of such groups must have access to correct information to avoid promulgating inaccurate theories and solutions. Group members benefit from the sharing of experiences, advice, information, and support. Berkun (1986) noted that women in a health collective and menopause rap groups at a women's center profited enormously from sharing their experiences and hearing about the experiences of other women.

Case 3

As Ms. C approached her menopause, she began to look for sources of support and information. Although her husband was a caring individual, she did not wish to complain to him constantly about her symptoms and fears. She was also not sure that he could understand how disruptive some of her menopausal symptoms could be. She had a good relationship with her physician but often felt somewhat hurried at her visits there. She was also concerned that he might put too much emphasis on taking hormone replacement therapy.

Ms. C saw an advertisement for a self-help group aimed at perimenopausal women and began attending this group on a weekly basis. Sessions lasted for 2 hours and involved information sharing as well as opportunities to discuss feelings and concerns about menopause. Ms. C was able to learn about a variety of approaches that the other participants had used to deal with menopausal symptoms. She also enjoyed the fellowship and opportunity to discuss her feelings and share her concerns and ideas with women in a similar situation.

Ms. C attended on a weekly basis for 8 weeks and then would drop in approximately once a month for another year. She found that as she went through menopause, she was able to reassure premenopausal women that their fears were not justified. She enjoyed this role of assisting other women in handling this period of their lives.

In some countries, self-support for menopausal women is better established than in other countries. In the Netherlands, a group called Vrouwen in de Overgang (VIDO) grew from a small support group of menopausal women to a program that exists in every city and town. VIDO not only provides support groups but also maintains a house in the country where midlife women can go to spend quiet weekends away from the stress of family or work. Members of this group also routinely talk about menopause to medical students (Cobb 1990).

Cobb (1990) developed a support network for menopausal women, which takes the form of a monthly bulletin—*A Friend Indeed*—that includes reports on developments in research about menopause, discussions of life events that occur at midlife, and advice about taking better care of themselves. Issues discussed include heart care, breast health, arthritis, migraine headaches, nutrition, exercise, anxiety, and depression.

Conclusion

D. M. McLaren and R. S. Breakey ("Self-Care Resource Corner: Its Impact on Appropriate Health Service Utilization," unpublished manuscript, Ann Arbor, University of Michigan, 1981) found that inappropriate use of health care service adds to escalating health care costs and impedes the effective and efficient provision of medical care. Group programs for menopausal women are cost-effective ways to help those women who experience physical and emotional distress around this midlife change. A limited number of women may require the intensive type of experience available in psychotherapeutically oriented groups or individual therapy. Many more could benefit from open-ended support groups, which allow women to share their experiences. Educational groups combining education about both the physical and psychological changes of menopause and the available treatment options are effective ways of reducing menopausal concerns and enhancing primary prevention of distressing menopausal symptoms. This approach also focuses on the woman as a proactive consumer of health services and allows her to make an informed selection from a wide variety of health care services and providers and to explore her options and choices (McElmurry and Huddleston 1991). Educational groups for women at midlife also provide the opportunity to enhance preventive health care skills, improve quality of life, and thereby decrease the number of menopausal and postmenopausal women afflicted with chronic disease (Bachmann 1990).

References

Abraham S, Perz J, Clarkson R, et al: Australian women's perceptions of hormone replacement therapy over 10 years. Maturitas 21:91–95, 1995

Anderson E, Hamburger S, Liu JH: Characteristics of menopausal women seeking assistance. Am J Obstet Gynecol 156:428–433, 1987

Avis NE, McKinley SM: A longitudinal analysis of women's attitudes towards the menopause: results from the Massachusetts Women's Health Study. Maturitas 13:65–79, 1991

Bachmann GA: The ideals of optional care for women at mid-life. Ann N Y Acad Sci 592:253–255, 1990

Ballinger CB: Psychiatric aspects of menopause. Br J Psychiatry 156:773–787, 1990

Berkun CS: In behalf of women over 40: understanding the importance of the menopause. Soc Work 31:378–384, 1986

Bowles CL: The menopausal experience: sociocultural influences and theoretical models, in The Meanings of Menopause: Historical, Medical and Clinical Perspectives. Edited by Formanek R. Hillsdale, NJ, Analytic Press, 1990, pp 157–175

Caplan G: Mastery of stress: psychosocial aspects. Am J Psychiatry 138:413–420, 1981

Cobb JO: Education of community and health care providers. Ann N Y Acad Sci 592:221–227, 1990

Dennerstein L: Psychiatric aspects of the climacteric, in The Menopause. Edited by Studd JWW, Whitehead MI. Oxford, UK, Blackwell Scientific, 1988, pp 43–54

Gath D, Iles S: Depression and the menopause. BMJ 300:1287–1288, 1990

Hamburger S, Anderson ER: The value of education and social-psychological support in a menopause clinic, in Multidisciplinary Perspectives on Menopause. Edited by Flint M, Kronenberg F, Utian W. New York, The New York Academy of Sciences, 1990, pp 242–249

Holte A, Mikkelsen A: Psychosocial determinants of climacteric complaints. Maturitas 13:205–215, 1991

La Rocco SA, Polit DF: Women's knowledge about menopause. Nurs Res 29:10–13, 1980

Lock M: Contested meanings of the menopause. Lancet 337:1270–1272, 1991

McElmurry BJ, Huddleston DS: Self-care and menopause: critical review of research. Health Care for Women International 12:15–26, 1991

Randall T: Women need more and better information on menopause from their physicians, says survey. JAMA 270:1664, 1993

Roberts PJ: The menopause and hormone replacement therapy: views of women in general practice receiving hormone replacement therapy. Br J Gen Pract 41:421–424, 1991

Stewart DE, Boydell K, Derzko C, et al: Psychologic distress during the menopausal years in women attending a menopause clinic. Int J Psychiatry Med 22:213–220, 1992

Stirtzinger R, Robinson GE, Crawford B: Educational approach to menopausal distress. Can Fam Physician 38:285–290, 1992

Weiss B: From workplace to community: an educational support program for menopause in transition, in The Modern Management of the Menopause: A Perspective for the 21st Century. Edited by Berg G, Hammar M. New York, Parthenon Publishing Group, 1994, pp 83–90

CHAPTER 11

Psychopharmacology

Margaret F. Jensvold, M.D.

As the population in general is aging, questions arise as to the appropriate treatment of psychological symptoms in female patients age 40–60 years—hormone replacement therapy (HRT), psychotropic medication, or both? For patients already taking psychotropic medications, will perimenopause or menopause have any effect on their need for or tolerance of psychotropic medications? Are there drug interactions between HRT and other drugs used to treat menopause and psychotropic medications that should be taken into account? In this chapter, I examine several topics relevant to clinicians, researchers, and health care consumers in understanding the relationships between menopause and psychopharmacology.

Menopause-Associated Medications for Treatment of Psychiatric Symptoms

Methodological issues in the menopause research available to date contribute to difficulty drawing conclusions about psychological symptoms in menopause and their treatment. These issues include the following (Stewart 1994):

- Populations studied in community-based population surveys and clinical studies are very different.

- Reliability of the diagnosis of menopausal state varies considerably with diagnostic method used—age alone, changes in menstrual status, or hormone levels.
- Some studies do not distinguish whether the subjects are perimenopausal (the period immediately preceding menopause and 1 year after the last menses) or postmenopausal (more than 12 months after the last menses).
- Many studies fail to indicate whether subjects are taking HRT or which types of HRT are used.
- Proportions of study populations found to have psychiatric illness vary considerably with the diagnostic method used—diagnostic interview or standardized psychometric instruments.
- Age and time since menopause are confounding variables that require sophisticated analyses to avoid methodological biases (Greendale et al. 1995).

In general, women take more medications, take more multiple medications, and appear to have more adverse effects from medications than men do, even when corrected for the numbers of medications taken (Baum et al. 1988). This highlights the importance of understanding sex differences, including those in midlife, in the need for and response to drugs.

Hormone Replacement Therapy or Psychotropic Medications for Treatment of Psychological Symptoms Common in the Perimenopause

Although the consensus of research appears to be that depression is not more common postmenopausally, high proportions of women presenting for treatment of perimenopausal symptoms have varying degrees of depression or other mild psychological symptoms.

Abundant basic scientific evidence indicates that estrogen has myriad effects on central nervous system (CNS) neurotransmitter systems, including the dopaminergic system, neuropeptides, gamma-aminobutyric acid (GABA), and the cholinergic system (McEwen 1994). Catecholestrogens, which are formed from estrogen in various brain sites, act on various receptors, including noradrenergic receptors, potentially influencing the monoamine system in a generalized or specific way (Smith 1994b). Various types of evidence indicate that estrogen has a general CNS excitatory effect (Smith 1994a), which could be interpreted as generally positive CNS effects. To what extent and in which patients exogenous estrogen is clinically useful for ameliorating psychological symptoms are still being determined.

Research to date indicates that when a peri- or postmenopausal patient's symptoms meet criteria for an affective disorder, HRT cannot be counted on to treat the affective disorder. For patients with milder symptoms, perhaps a subsyndromal state, it is not always readily apparent whether the patient should be treated with HRT, psychotropic medication, or both. A conservative approach would be to treat with HRT, determine to what extent the symptoms resolve with HRT (or are worsened by HRT), and then decide about psychotropic medication based on the remaining symptoms. Personal psychiatric history, family history, and severity and duration of symptoms help to determine whether psychotropic medication should be instituted.

A topic about which little has been written, but clinical observations have been made, is that panic attacks and hot flashes may be difficult to distinguish in some patients, either patients with long-standing panic disorder or patients with a question of new-onset panic. Treatment with estrogen replacement therapy (ERT) may be necessary to help distinguish between hot flashes and panic. Hot flashes would be ameliorated by ERT, whereas panic may be unaffected or worsened by ERT. Case reports of panic disorder induced by ERT (Dembert et al. 1994) and onset of panic in the latter half of pregnancy (Griez et al. 1995) are consistent with a panicogenic effect of estrogen.

Another topic about which little has been written is that some peri- and postmenopausal patients who completed daily symptom ratings continued to document regular cyclical mood changes similar to their earlier premenstrual mood changes for more than a year after cessation of menses (Dalton 1977). Assuming this is not an expectancy effect, it may indicate continued cycling of the "endogenous time clock" within the CNS (Jensvold 1996a) for some time after the cessation of catamenial ovarian activity in some peri- and postmenopausal women. Whether pharmacological treatment (e.g., antidepressant medication) used to treat the patient's premenstrual dysphoric disorder should be continued has yet to be studied.

In reality, whether a patient is treated with HRT or psychotropic medication is often determined by which specialist she sees. Psychiatrists generally do not prescribe hormonal medications, and some may be unlikely to evaluate the hormonal status of the patient or to refer the patient to a gynecologist, internist, or family doctor. Although most psychotropic medications are prescribed by physicians other than psychiatrists, nonpsychiatrists are likely to follow up patients' psychiatric conditions less closely and are likely to have less time to talk with or listen to patients than psychiatrists do. These facts alone are likely to contribute to many patients being overtreated, undertreated, or otherwise not correctly treated. Patients would benefit from psychiatrists who learn how to evaluate peri- and postmenopausal status, learn how to discuss the relative merits of HRT (Lerner 1995), and develop sources of referral for HRT.

Estrogen for Treatment of Dementia

Estrogen is not currently a standard accepted treatment for dementia. However, evidence from a variety of human and animal studies involving the cholinergic system, memory, and dementia (reviewed by Ohkura et al. 1994 and others) suggested that estrogen may eventually become part of the pharmacological armamentarium for the prevention and/or treatment of dementia.

Estrogen administration is associated with increases in synthesis and activity of choline acetyltransferase (ChAT), a key enzyme involved in the synthesis of acetylcholine, the neurotransmitter considered most important in dementia (Kaufman et al. 1988). ERT has been associated with improvements in memory in postmenopausal women (Furuhjelm and Fedor-Freybergh 1976) and surgically menopausal women (Sherwin 1988). Estrogen treatment of patients with dementia of the Alzheimer's type resulted in improvements in psychometric testing results, cerebral blood flow, and electroencephalogram findings (Ohkura et al. 1994). (For more information, see Shapiro, Chapter 7, and Charney and Stewart, Chapter 8, in this volume.)

Combination Estrogen-Testosterone for Treatment of Sexual Dysfunction

Testosterone, either orally or in depot pellet form, added to ERT is often successful in restoring sexual desire, sexual function, and a sense of well-being to naturally menopausal (Studd et al. 1977) and surgically menopausal (Sherwin and Gelfand 1987) women (see also Lamont, Chapter 5, in this volume). Masculinizing side effects, however, may result in some women.

"Iatrogenic Premenstrual Syndrome"

HRT can cause an iatrogenic psychiatric condition resembling premenstrual dysphoric disorder because the progesterone component of cyclic replacement therapy sometimes causes symptoms during the progesterone treatment phase or during the "pill-free interval" immediately following the progesterone phase (Hammarback et al. 1985; Whitehead 1983). The symptoms can often be ameliorated by reducing the progestogen dose. Whitehead found that approximately 10% of patients experienced a premenstrual-like syndrome after taking 500 µg/day of norgestrel added to estrogen therapy. The frequency and severity of symptoms decreased when the norgestrel dosage was reduced to 150 µg/day (Whitehead 1983).

Dennerstein (1991) pointed out that the type of progestogen may also have an effect, because studies with 19-norsteroids have reported more adverse psychological effects than those with oral micronized progesterone (De Lignieres and Vincens 1982; Hammarback et al. 1985). In addition to lowering the progestogen dose or switching to a different progestogen, changing to continuous combined HRT or "long-cyclic" HRT (pill-free interval occurring only every 3 or 4 months) (David et al. 1994) can be helpful. Individual patient vulnerability factors may also play a role. It has been suggested that histories of premenstrual dysphoria or postpartum depression may be predictive, although this has not been studied.

Treatments for Common Perimenopausal Symptoms

In population-based studies conducted in North America, Europe, and Australia, the proportions of postmenopausal women taking HRT have ranged from 3% (Italy) to 32% (California) (Harris et al. 1990; Oddens et al. 1992). With the majority of eligible women not taking HRT, a large industry has grown up around over-the-counter combination preparations and natural food or herbal treatments for menopause (Kronenberg 1995; Notelovitz 1994). Most of these remedies are untested with regard to their efficacy for treatment of menopausal symptoms and, more specifically, the psychological symptoms that may accompany menopause. Some of the most commonly used include ginkgo, quon do, ginseng, and vitamin E. Some foods, including flax and soy products, contain phytoestrogens, a nonsteroid form of estrogen, and are used in a dietary approach to treatment of menopausal symptoms. Some women who have been told by medical professionals that they cannot take estrogen because of medical contraindications have self-prescribed herbal and/or dietary preparations containing phytoestrogens. The extent to which nonsteroid estrogens produce untoward medical or psychological effects comparable to those of steroid estrogens has not been studied.

Controlled trials of alternative treatments for menopausal symptoms are beginning to be reported. Acupuncture and relaxation therapy (Wyon et al. 1995) have decreased hot flashes in controlled trials. High response rates to placebo, with placebo effects lasting at least 3 months, highlight the need for well-controlled trials (Kronenberg 1995). (For more information on alternative treatments, see Chapter 7.)

Gonadotropin-Releasing Hormone Agonists

Potent gonadotropin-releasing hormone (GnRH) agonists are not used to *treat* menopause but rather are being used increasingly frequently to induce a temporary, reversible menopausal state in some reproductive-age women, including some patients with severe premenstrual psychological symptoms (Hammarback and Backstrom

1988). Inducing a reversible menopausal state will test whether the menopausal state alleviates menstrual cycle–related symptoms without the permanency or invasiveness of ovariectomy. Symptoms that are tightly linked to the menstrual cycle are most likely to be alleviated by GnRH agonist therapy. Some cases have been reported of affective syndromes becoming unentrained from the menstrual cycle during GnRH agonist treatment. Hypoestrogenic symptoms due to GnRH agonists may be managed by adding low-dose HRT or clonidine. Serial bone scans are required to monitor for development of osteoporosis.

Drug Interactions Between Menopause-Associated Medications and Psychotropic Medications

With many women age 40 and older taking, or considering taking, both menopause-associated and psychotropic medications, questions are bound to arise about whether drug interactions are of concern. Drug interactions of oral contraceptives have been reviewed a number of times (e.g., Geurts et al. 1993; Jensvold 1996b). However, very little has been written about interactions between HRT and other drugs. What is known about drug interactions of oral contraceptives cannot be assumed to apply to HRT. The doses and potency of hormones in HRT approximate those of the endogenous sex steroid hormones of reproductive-age women. Blood levels with sequential HRT tend to mimic the normal menstrual cycle, whereas continuous therapy approximates an anovulatory cycle (Sitruk-Ware 1991). In contrast, the hormone levels achieved with oral contraceptives greatly exceed those of the normal menstrual cycle, and the synthetic hormones used in oral contraceptives generally have much greater potency than natural forms of the hormones typically used in HRT. The little that is known of the effects of the normal menstrual cycle on drugs (Jensvold 1996a) may be more relevant to understanding drug interactions of HRT than information about drug interactions of oral contraceptives.

In the following sections, I review drug interactions of medications commonly taken in relation to menopause, with emphasis on interactions with psychotropic medications.

Replacement Estrogen

Tricyclic Antidepressants

Toxicity. Studies reporting increased side effects with estrogen–tricyclic antidepressant combinations have all involved oral contraceptives rather than HRT. Khurana (1972) reported the case of a 32-year-old woman taking 2.5–7.5 mg of conjugated estrogen (much more than is typically used in HRT today) and 100 mg of imipramine. The patient's long-term side effects of extreme lethargy, nausea, constant headaches, and low-normal blood pressure eventually led to hospitalization. The side effects resolved when estrogen was stopped.

Prange and Wilson (Editor 1972) administered either placebo, imipramine plus 25 or 50 μg/day of ethinyl estradiol (the amounts used in low-dose oral contraceptives), or imipramine plus placebo to 30 depressed women for 2 weeks. The subjects taking the imipramine-estradiol combination experienced more side effects, including drowsiness, tremor, and hypotension, than the other groups but also more therapeutic benefit in this brief trial.

In a retrospective study of subjects taking various types of oral contraceptives and clomipramine, no increased toxicity or effectiveness of clomipramine was found (Beaumont 1973).

Akathisia. Three cases have been reported of akathisia developing with the combination of conjugated estrogens (used in HRT) and tricyclic antidepressants (Krishnan et al. 1984). Two women taking conjugated estrogens for years since hysterectomy and oophorectomy developed akathisia within hours of starting amitriptyline. Akathisia resolved when amitriptyline was discontinued. A 24-year-old woman was given clomipramine and conjugated estrogens simultaneously. Akathisia developed over the course of a week and resolved when conjugated estrogen was discontinued.

Metabolism effects. A study of single doses of imipramine administered to women taking low-dose-estrogen oral contraceptives and to control women not taking oral contraceptives found little change in imipramine kinetics after intravenous dosing but increased bioavailability with increased apparent clearance and increased half-life after oral dosing (Abernethy et al. 1984). The findings were consistent with the estrogen in oral contraceptives inhibiting hepatic oxidation of imipramine.

Animal studies indicate that estrogenic compounds may impair the metabolism of imipramine (Tephly and Mannering 1968).

Recommendations.   It has been recommended in reproductive-age women taking oral contraceptives that tricyclic antidepressants be given at low doses and increased gradually, monitoring for side effects. The tricyclic antidepressant–oral contraceptive combination prescribed in this way is considered safe (Ciraulo et al. 1995). Similar recommendations would be expected to render the tricyclic antidepressant–HRT combination safe as well.

Hepatic Microsomal Enzyme-Inducing Agents

Because estrogen is metabolized mainly via the liver, by the cytochrome P450 system, it is presumed that all microsomal enzyme-inducing agents could cause lower than expected estrogen levels. Such agents include some anticonvulsants (carbamazepine, phenytoin, and primidone), barbiturates, phenylbutazone (nonsteroidal anti-inflammatory drug), and rifampin (antibiotic).

Phenytoin and carbamazepine are known to alter single-dose pharmacokinetics of ethinyl estradiol (Crawford et al. 1990). Patients taking these anticonvulsants may need increased doses of oral contraceptives.

One case report involved HRT. A 24-year-old woman had taken 1.25 mg of conjugated estrogen for 2 years since hysterectomy and oophorectomy (Notelovitz et al. 1981). When 300 mg/day of phenytoin was added for treatment of suspected seizures, her hot flashes resumed, estrogen levels decreased, and gonadotropin levels became elevated. After phenytoin was discontinued, follow-up estrogen and gonadotropin levels indicated adequate estrogen replacement on the same dose of conjugated estrogens. The authors pointed out that as lower doses of estrogen are used, clinically significant interactions between estrogens and phenytoin or other hepatic enzyme-inducing agents are more likely to occur.

Monitoring the clinical benefit from replacement estrogen, measuring the serum estradiol levels if necessary, and increasing the estrogen dosage when appropriate should make the combination of replacement estrogen with hepatic enzyme-inducing agents safe. Switching to medications that do not induce hepatic microsomal enzymes will be the option of choice in some cases. For example, the mood stabilizers valproate and lithium do not induce hepatic microsomal enzymes and thus would be expected to have less effect on replacement estrogen than carbamazepine does.

Ethinyl estradiol, the form of estrogen most commonly used in HRT, is metabolized in the liver by 2-hydroxylation by cytochrome P450 3A4 (also called CY P450 NF) (Goldzieher 1994; Guengerich 1988). Although the major degradative pathway of ethinyl estradiol involves cytochrome P450 3A4 (Guengerich 1988), there is some suggestion that cytochrome P450 1A2 (Goldzieher 1994) and cytochrome P450 2C8 (Back and Orme 1994; Goldzieher 1994) may also be involved in oxidative metabolism of ethinyl estradiol. Cytochromes P450 3A4, 1A2, and 2C influence the oxidative metabolism of some psychotropic and other drugs (see Table 11–1). Although interactions between ethinyl estradiol and the drugs whose metabolism is affected by cytochromes P450 3A4, 1A2, and 2C are possible, the clinical significance of such drug interactions is not known. Fluoxetine, norfluoxetine, sertraline, and paroxetine are potent inhibitors of cytochrome P450 2D6 (Nemeroff et al. 1996). Cytochrome P450 2D6 has not been reported to influence metabolism of ethinyl estradiol.

Dantrolene

Hepatotoxicity has occurred more frequently in women older than 35 years taking estrogen and dantrolene (Drug Facts and Comparisons 1996). Relevancy to menopause or HRT is not clear.

Smoking

Decreased estrogen effect may occur with smoking as a result of increased estrogen metabolism (Jensen et al. 1985). Avoiding concurrent use is recommended.

Table 11–1. Psychotropic drugs with metabolism associated with cytochrome P450 1A2, 2C, and 3A4

1A2
Drugs whose oxidative metabolism is associated with CY P450 1A2
Amitriptyline
Caffeine
Clomipramine
Clozapine
Fluvoxamine
Haloperidol
Imipramine
Verapamil

CY P450 1A2 is inhibited by
Fluvoxamine

CY P450 1A2 is implicated in drug interactions with
Clozapine
Theophylline

2C
Drugs whose oxidative metabolism is associated with CY P450 2C
Amitriptyline
Clomipramine
Diazepam
Hexobarbital
Mephobarbital
Phenytoin

Drugs believed to inhibit CY P450 2C
Fluoxetine
Fluvoxamine
Sertraline

3A4
Drugs whose oxidative metabolism is associated with CY P450 3A4
Amitriptyline
Alprazolam
Carbamazepine
Clomipramine
Dexamethasone
Imipramine
Midazolam
Nefazodone
Sertraline
Triazolam
Verapamil

Plasma concentrations of the drugs immediately above have increased when administered with
Fluoxetine
Fluvoxamine
Nefazodone
Sertraline

Source. Modified from Nemeroff et al. 1996.

Corticosteroids

Four of five studies (e.g., Legler and Benet 1986) have reported that enhanced efficacy or increased toxicity of corticosteroids occurs with concurrent estrogen use in oral contraceptive users. The clinical significance is not established, and it is not clear whether this finding has any relevance to HRT users.

Replacement Progestogen

Tricyclic Antidepressants

Norethindrone, a progestogen used in oral contraceptives, inhibited metabolism of imipramine in mice (Bellward et al. 1974).

Hepatic Microsomal Enzyme-Inducing Agents

Progesterone, like ethinyl estradiol, is metabolized by the hepatic cytochrome P450 enzyme system (Ciraulo et al. 1995). Several hepatic microsomal enzyme-inducing agents, including carbamazepine (Crawford et al. 1990) and rifampin, decreased serum progesterone levels in subjects taking oral contraceptives.

Several progestogens used in oral contraceptives are potent inactivators of cytochrome P450 3A4. In decreasing order of potency, they are gestodene, 3-ketodesogestrel, norethindrone, and levonorgestrel (Sillem and Teichmann 1994). The relation to medroxyprogesterone acetate, the progestogen commonly used in HRT, is not known.

No studies of hepatic enzyme-inducing agents affecting HRT have been reported. A theoretical concern is that hepatic enzyme-inducing agents could decrease the effectiveness of progesterone in HRT. Patients should be monitored for clinical efficacy of progesterone in HRT (with sequential combined HRT, regular bleeding should occur; with continuous combined HRT, bleeding should not occur after an initial period of irregular bleeding). If low progesterone levels are suspected, progesterone levels may be measured and/or the progesterone dose may be increased.

Replacement Testosterone or Methyltestosterone

Interactions between the psychotropic medications and the androgens used in HRT, testosterone and methyltestosterone, have not been reported.

We are not aware of reports of hepatic cytochrome enzyme effects on testosterone or interactions with testosterone.

Clonidine

Clonidine, a centrally acting α_2-adrenergic agonist, ameliorates hot flashes in some women.

β-Blockers

Numerous reports (e.g., Lilja et al. 1980; Vernon and Sakula 1979) document that the rebound hypertensive response that typically follows clonidine withdrawal is enhanced by β-blockers. Paradoxical hypertensive response *during* treatment with clonidine and propranolol has also been reported.

Tricyclic Antidepressants

Tricyclic antidepressants have been reported to decrease the antihypertensive effect of clonidine (i.e., tricyclic antidepressants may make clonidine a less effective antihypertensive agent) (Van Spanning and van Zwieten 1973). For perimenopausal women who are not hypertensive and are taking clonidine for hot flashes, this interaction may be potentially beneficial. For patients with hypertension, hot flashes, and depression, treatment with clonidine for hot flashes and an antidepressant other than a tricyclic antidepressant should be considered.

Other Psychotropic Drugs

Other psychotropic drugs with reported interactions with clonidine include levodopa (decreased levodopa effect), naloxone (naloxone may decrease the effect of clonidine, possibly via release of endogenous CNS opioids), phenothiazines (organic brain syndrome) (Allen and Flemenbaum 1979), and verapamil (two cases of atrioventricular block) (Jaffe et al. 1994).

Alendronate

No drug interactions have yet been reported for alendronate, a biphosphonate that prevents postmenopausal osteoporosis.

Age and Menopause Effects on Drugs

Differences in prescribing medications for postmenopausal elderly women compared with younger women may be attributed to the physiology of aging, physiology of disease, high numbers of concurrent medications, and social context of illness and treatment (Salzman et al. 1995). The relative contributions of these factors may be difficult to distinguish at times. Although significant heterogeneity exists in the aging process, several commonalities are seen (Dubovsky 1994; Salzman et al. 1995).

Although menopause is often a reminder to the woman that she is getting older, the onset of menopause and elderly status occur at different ages. The average age at onset of menopause is 50, and the usual age cutoff for drug studies of the elderly population compared with younger populations is 65. Age and menopause effects are often confounded in pharmacological research. First, I summarize current knowledge of age effects on drugs and then review menopause effects.

Pharmacokinetics refers to the delivery of the drug to and from the site of action (e.g., absorption, bioavailability, metabolism, clearance, and excretion). Pharmacodynamics refers to the effects of the drug at the site of action (e.g., receptor binding, receptor populations and sensitivity, second-messenger effects, genomic effects).

Age Effects

Several recent reviews examined the topic of age effects on drugs (e.g., Dubovsky 1994; Salzman et al. 1995; please refer to these reviews for details).

In summary, gastrointestinal absorption is not decreased in the elderly, but some drugs commonly taken by the elderly (antacids and anticholinergic drugs) delay absorption of other medications. Hepatic blood flow decreases with age, resulting in slowed first-pass metabolism and therefore increased blood levels of some drugs. Metabolism producing biologically active metabolites (called *phase I metabolism*) is slowed with aging, resulting in longer half-lives and higher blood levels of many medications.

Fatty tissue increases as a proportion of body weight with age, and the proportion of body weight that is water decreases. Most psychotropic medications are lipophilic (lithium is the notable exception, being hydrophilic), which means that psychotropic medications (other than lithium) will stay in the body longer, will take longer to equilibrate, and may take longer to achieve either therapeutic benefit or side effects (Abernethy 1992). Renal blood flow decreases with age, decreasing creatinine clearance and contributing to longer half-lives of drugs and higher blood levels.

Changes in brain structure with age, such as loss of neurons, contribute to increased sensitivity to a variety of side effects of medications, including particularly sedative, psychomotor, orthostatic, and anticholinergic effects. Dubovsky (1994) cautioned, however, that no evidence exists for the common assumption of increased sensitivity to beneficial effects of medication with aging. Decreased sensitivity of β-adrenergic receptors, benzodiazepine receptors, and other receptors may contribute to decreased efficacy of some drugs in the elderly.

The cumulative effects of the pharmacokinetic changes with age tend to be slower absorption, longer time to reach steady state, larger volume of distribution for lipophilic drugs (most psychotropic drugs, except lithium), slower excretion, and longer half-lives (Dubovsky 1994). On the other hand, the great interindividual hetereogeneity in rates of metabolism means that some elderly patients need the same doses that are used in younger patients. Pharmacodynamic changes appear to increase sensitivity to side effects while possibly decreasing effectiveness of some drugs in the elderly.

Menopause Effects

The variables of sex (the biological category of male or female) and gender (a biopsychosocially constructed variable) often have been overlooked as critical variables in drug studies. The effects of menopause on drugs have rarely been addressed. Hamilton and Yonkers (1996; Yonkers and Hamilton 1996) reviewed the research to date on menopause effects on drugs.

In summary, some evidence indicates that gastric emptying time is affected by menopause, but effects are different for liquids compared with solids and fatty liquids. Gastric acid secretion appears to be somewhat affected by menopause (increased) and by conjugated estrogens (decreased). Cerebral blood flow declines in the peri- and postmenopausal years, whereas replacement estrogen increases cerebral blood flow (Ohkura et al. 1995). Levels of many serum proteins apparently change with menopause but not with a simple pattern that is readily generalizable. Evidence suggests that estrogen in oral contraceptives affects metabolism (glucuronidation, increased; hydroxylation and demethylation, decreased) and that progesterone increases glomerular filtration rate, but the relevance to menopause is less clear.

A fully integrated understanding of the effects of sex and age on drugs has yet to be achieved and will require additional research. But initial tentative conclusions are suggested by the limited information available to date. Hamilton and Yonkers (1996) concluded:

> [A]ge-related changes generally may not be as pronounced in women as in men. . . . Women of any age group have a larger proportion of adipose tissue and [volume of distribution] Vd compared with men. There is a strong age-related decline in total drug [clearance] CL in men, who tend to clear drugs faster when younger, such that with age they lose their more efficient disposition status relative to women (this may be an advantage or disadvantage, according to the situation); the effect of age in females is generally far less pronounced. . . . Effects of sex on absorption may be somewhat more important than those of age (age has negligible effects on absorption); however, hepatic metabolism and renal CL are often relatively more important than absorption. Particularly for hepatically biotransformed drugs, if doses were advisedly decreased somewhat in young women compared with young men, then there might be relatively little need to decrease dosages *further* in older women. Instead, it appears that age transforms the needs of older *men* (with slower CL than younger men) to more closely match those of younger *women* (also with slower CL than younger men). (pp. 37–38)

The Future

Several current trends in pharmacology research promise to increase the future understanding of psychopharmacology and the menopause. These include

- Breakthroughs in the understanding of the basic biology of sex steroids, particularly neurosteroids (neuroactive endogenous steroids and steroid metabolites in the CNS) (Smith 1994b)
- Increases in attention to pharmacodynamics, which have had to be preceded by increased understanding of pharmacokinetics (Jensvold et al. 1996)
- Research on the effects of sex steroids on mood, anxiety, and cognition and on drug metabolism, interactions, and effectiveness
- Research on alternative treatments for menopausal symptoms (Kronenberg 1995; Notelovitz 1994; Wyon et al. 1995)
- Publication of the U.S. Food and Drug Administration's (FDA) guidelines for studies of HRT (FDA HRT Working Group 1995) and recent FDA guidelines recommending that women and the elderly be included in drug development studies and that data be analyzed to examine for sex and age differences in drugs (Jensvold et al. 1996; Merkatz et al. 1993; U.S. Food and Drug Administration 1993).

References

Abernethy DR: Psychotropic drugs and the aging process: pharmacokinetics and pharmacodynamics, in Clinical Geriatric Psychiatry, 2nd Edition. Edited by Salzman C. Baltimore, MD, Williams & Wilkins, 1992, pp 61–76

Abernethy DR, Greenblatt DJ, Shader RI: Imipramine disposition in users of oral contraceptive steroids. Clin Pharmacol Ther 35:792–797, 1984

Allen RM, Flemenbaum A: Delirium associated with combined fluphenazine–clonidine therapy. J Clin Psychiatry 40:236–237, 1979

Back DJ, Orme MLE: Drug interactions, in Pharmacology of the Contraceptive Steroids. Edited by Goldzieher JW, Fotherby K. New York, Raven, 1994, pp 127–141

Baum C, Kennedy D, Knapp DE, et al: Prescription drug use in 1984 and changes over time. Med Care 26:105–114, 1988

Beaumont G: Drug interactions with clomipramine (Anafranil). J Int Med Res 1:480–484, 1973

Bellward GD, Morgan RG, Szombathy VH: The effects of pretreatment of mice with norethindrone on the metabolism in [14C]-imipramine by the liver microsomal drug–metabolizing enzymes. Can J Physiol Pharmacol 52:28–38, 1974

Ciraulo DA, Shader RI, Greenblatt DJ, et al: Drug Interactions in Psychiatry, 2nd Edition. Baltimore, MD, Williams & Wilkins, 1995

Crawford P, Chadwick DJ, Martin C, et al: The interaction of phenytoin and carbamazepine with combined oral contraceptive steroids. Br J Clin Pharmacol 30:892–896, 1990

Dalton K: The Premenstrual Syndrome and Progesterone Therapy. Chicago, IL, Year Book Medical Publishers, 1977

David A, Czernobilsky B, Weisglass L: Long-cyclic hormonal therapy in postmenopausal women, in The Modern Management of the Menopause: A Perspective for the 21st Century. Edited by Berg G, Hammar M. New York, Parthenon Publishing, 1994, pp 463–470

De Lignieres B, Vincens M: Differential effects of exogenous oestradiol and progesterone on mood in post-menopausal women; individual dose/effect relationship. Maturitas 4:67–72, 1982

Dembert ML, Dinneen MP, Opsahl MS: Estrogen-induced panic disorder (letter). Am J Psychiatry 151:1246, 1994

Dennerstein L: Mood and menopause, in The Menopause and Hormonal Replacement Therapy: Facts and Controversies. Edited by Sitruk-Ware R, Utian WH. New York, Marcel Dekker, 1991, pp 101–118

Drug Facts and Comparisons, 1996 Edition. St. Louis, MO, Facts and Comparisons, 1996

Dubovsky SL: Geriatric neuropsychopharmacology, in The American Psychiatric Press Textbook of Geriatric Neuropsychiatry. Edited by Coffey CE, Cummings JL, Lovell MR, et al. Washington, DC, American Psychiatric Press, 1994, pp 596–631

Editor: Estrogen may well affect response to antidepressant (editorial). JAMA 219:143–144, 1972

FDA HRT Working Group: Guidance for clinical evaluation of combination estrogen/progestin–containing drug products used for hormone replacement therapy of postmenopausal women. Menopause 2(3):131–136, 1995

Furuhjelm M, Fedor-Freybergh P: The influence of estrogens on the psyche in climacteric and post-menopausal women, in Consensus on Menopause Research. Edited by Van Keep PA, Greenblatt RB, Albeaux-Fernet MM. Baltimore, MD, Park Press, 1976, pp 84–93

Geurts TBP, Goorissen EM, Sitsen JMA: Summary of Drug Interactions With Oral Contraceptives. New York, Parthenon Publishing, 1993

Goldzieher JW: Pharmacokinetics and metabolism of ethynyl estrogens, in Pharmacology of the Contraceptive Steroids. Edited by Goldzieher JW, Fotherby K. New York, Raven, 1994, pp 127–141

Greendale GA, Hogan P, Kritz-Silverstein D, et al: Age at menopause in women participating in the Postmenopausal Estrogen/Progestins Interventions (PEPI) Trial: an example of bias introduced by selection criteria. Menopause 2(1):27–34, 1995

Griez EJL, Hauzer R, Meijer J: Pregnancy and estrogen-induced panic. Am J Psychiatry 152:1688, 1995

Guengerich FP: Oxidation of 17-alpha-ethinylestradiol by human liver cytochrome P-450. Mol Pharmacol 33:500–508, 1988

Hamilton JA, Yonkers KA: Sex differences in pharmacokinetics of psychotropic medications, part I: physiological basis for effects, in Psychopharmacology and Women: Sex, Gender, and Hormones. Edited by Jensvold MF, Halbreich U, Hamilton JA. Washington, DC, American Psychiatric Press, 1996, pp 11–42

Hammarback S, Backstrom T: Induced anovulation as treatment of premenstrual tension syndrome. Acta Obstet Gynecol Scand 67:159–166, 1988

Hammarback S, Backstrom T, Holst J, et al: Cyclical mood changes as in the premenstrual syndrome during sequential estrogen-progestogen postmenopausal replacement therapy. Acta Obstet Gynecol Scand 64:393–397, 1985

Harris RB, Laws A, Reddy VM, et al: Are women using postmenopausal estrogens? A community survey. Am J Public Health 80:1266–1268, 1990

Jaffe R, Livshits T, Bursztyn M: Adverse interaction between clonidine and verapamil. Ann Pharmacother 28:881–883, 1994

Jensen J, Christiansen C, Rodbro P: Cigarette smoking, serum estrogens, and bone loss during hormone-replacement therapy early after menopause. N Engl J Med 313:973–975, 1985

Jensvold MF: Nonpregnant reproductive-age women, part I: the menstrual cycle and psychopharmacology, in Psychopharmacology and Women: Sex, Gender, and Hormones. Edited by Jensvold MF, Halbreich U, Hamilton JA. Washington, DC, American Psychiatric Press, 1996a, pp 139–169

Jensvold MF: Nonpregnant reproductive-age women, part II: exogenous sex steroid hormones and psychopharmacology, in Psychopharmacology and Women: Sex, Gender, and Hormones. Edited by Jensvold MF, Halbreich U, Hamilton JA. Washington, DC, American Psychiatric Press, 1996b, pp 171–190

Jensvold MF, Hamilton JA, Halbreich U: Future research directions: methodological considerations for advancing gender-sensitive pharmacology, in Psychopharmacology and Women: Sex, Gender, and Hormones. Edited by Jensvold MF, Halbreich U, Hamilton JA. Washington, DC, American Psychiatric Press, 1996, pp 415–429

Kaufman H, Vadasz C, Lajtha A: Effects of estradiol and dexamethasone on choline acetyltransferase activity in various rat brain regions. Brain Res 453:389–392, 1988

Khurana RC: Estrogen-imipramine interaction. JAMA 222:702–703, 1972

Krishnan KR, France RD, Ellinwood EH: Tricyclic-induced akathisia in patients taking conjugated estrogens. Am J Psychiatry 141:696–697, 1984

Kronenberg F: Alternative therapies: new opportunities for menopause research. Menopause 2(1):1–2, 1995

Legler UF, Benet LZ: Marked alterations in dose-dependent prednisolone kinetics in women taking oral contraceptives. Clin Pharmacol Ther 39:425–429, 1986

Lerner S: Counseling the patient at menopause concerning hormone replacement therapy. Menopause 2(3):175–180, 1995

Lilja M, Jounela AJ, Juustila H, et al: Interaction of clonidine and beta-blockers. Acta Medica Scandinavia 207:173–176, 1980

McEwen BS: Ovarian steroids have diverse effects on brain structure and function, in The Modern Management of the Menopause: A Perspective for the 21st Century. Edited by Berg G, Hammar M. New York, Parthenon Publishing, 1994, pp 269–278

Merkatz RB, Temple R, Sobel S, et al: Inclusion of women in clinical trials—policies for population subgroups. N Engl J Med 329:288–296, 1993

Nemeroff CB, DeVane CL, Pollock BG: Newer antidepressants and the cytochrome P450 system. Am J Psychiatry 153:311–320, 1996

Notelovitz M: Non-hormonal management of the menopause, in The Modern Management of the Menopause: A Perspective for the 21st Century. Edited by Berg G, Hammar M. New York, Parthenon Publishing, 1994, pp 513–524

Notelovitz M, Tjapkes J, Ware M: Interaction between estrogen and Dilantin in a menopausal woman. N Engl J Med 304:788–789, 1981

Oddens BJ, Boulet MJ, Lehert P, et al: Has the climacteric been medicalized? A study of the use of medication for climacteric complaints in four countries. Maturitas 15:171–181, 1992

Ohkura T, Isse K, Akazawa K, et al: An open trial of estrogen therapy for dementia of the Alzheimer type in women, in The Modern Management of the Menopause: A Perspective for the 21st Century. Edited by Berg G, Hammar M. New York, Parthenon Publishing, 1994, pp 315–333

Ohkura T, Teshima Y, Isse K, et al: Estrogen increases cerebral and cerebellar blood flows in postmenopausal women. Menopause 2(1):13–18, 1995

Salzman C, Satlin A, Burrows AB: Geriatric psychopharmacology, in The American Psychiatric Press Textbook of Psychopharmacology. Edited by Schatzberg AF, Nemeroff CB. Washington, DC, American Psychiatric Press, 1995, pp 803–821

Sherwin BB: Estrogen and/or androgen replacement therapy and cognitive functioning in surgically menopausal women. Psychoneuroendocrinology 13:345–357, 1988

Sherwin BB, Gelfand MM: The role of androgen in the maintenance of sexual functioning in oophorectomized women. Psychosom Med 49:397–409, 1987

Sillem MH, Teichmann AT: The liver, in Pharmacology of the Contraceptive Steroids. Edited by Goldzieher JW, Fotherby K. New York, Raven, 1994, pp 247–257

Sitruk-Ware R: Hormonal replacement therapy: what to prescribe, how, and for how long, in The Menopause and Hormonal Replacement Therapy: Facts and Controversies. Edited by Sitruk-Ware R, Utian WH. New York, Marcel Dekker, 1991, pp 259–282

Smith SS: Activating effects of estradiol on brain activity, in The Modern Management of the Menopause: A Perspective for the 21st Century. Edited by Berg G, Hammar M. New York, Parthenon Publishing, 1994a, pp 279–294

Smith SS: Hormones, mood and neurobiology—a summary, in The Modern Management of the Menopause: A Perspective for the 21st Century. Edited by Berg G, Hammar M. New York, Parthenon Publishing, 1994b, pp 257–268

Stewart DE: Psychology of menopause. Paper presented at the annual meeting of the American Psychiatric Association, Philadelphia, PA, May 1994

Studd JWW, Collins WP, Chakravarti S: Oestradiol and testosterone implants in the treatment of psychosexual problems in the post-menopause. Br J Obstet Gynaecol 84:314–319, 1977

Tephly TR, Mannering GJ: Inhibition of drug metabolism vs. inhibition of drug metabolism by steroids. Mol Pharmacol 4:10–14, 1968

U.S. Food and Drug Administration: Guideline for the study and evaluation of gender differences in the clinical evaluation of drugs (U.S. Food and Drug Administration Docket No 93D-0236). Rockville, MD, 1993, pp 1–53

Van Spanning HW, van Zwieten PA: The interference of tricyclic antidepressants with the central hypotensive effect of clonidine. Eur J Pharmacol 24:402–404, 1973

Vernon C, Sakula A: Fatal rebound hypertension after abrupt withdrawal of clonidine and propranolol. Br J Clin Pract 33:112–121, 1979

Whitehead MI: The menopause, part A: hormone "replacement" therapy—the controversies, in Handbook of Psychosomatic Obstetrics and Gynecology. Edited by Dennerstein L, Burrows G. Amsterdam, Elsevier Biomedical Press, 1983, pp 445–481

Wyon Y, Lindgren R, Lundeberg T, et al: Effects of acupuncture on climacteric vasomotor symptoms, quality of life, and urinary excretion of neuropeptides among postmenopausal women. Menopause 2(1):3–12, 1995

Yonkers KA, Hamilton JA: Sex differences in pharmacokinetics of psychotropic medications, part II: effects on selected psychotropics, in Psychopharmacology and Women: Sex, Gender, and Hormones. Edited by Jensvold MF, Halbreich U, Hamilton JA. Washington, DC, American Psychiatric Press, 1996, pp 43–71

CHAPTER 12

Beyond Menopause:
Vulnerability Versus Hardiness

Susan Feldman, M.A.
Yael Netz, Ph.D.

How do I view ageing in general? It is a challenge, and I want to live to the fullest physically, mentally, emotionally and spiritually and enjoy every moment of my life. There are many slips from the ideal, but the goal of a full life is never lost. I do not often think of my ageing; the mirror of course reminds me of it. When I see the wrinkled, sagging skin of my face I tell myself that my skin is the time map of my life's experiences, it has its own values and beauty. It is uniquely mine.

Kamler and Feldman 1995

*T*he years beyond menopause have been viewed in a poor light, partially because of the dominance of the medically oriented biological decline model of aging and partially because of the prevalence of derogatory stereotypes regarding the elderly, in general, and women, in particular. Women are more likely than men to be penalized for aging because Western society is less tolerant of the aging process and its physical manifestations in women (Kuhn and Gray Panthers 1974; Markson 1994; Sontag 1972).

The reality is that for most older women, the years after the menopause are characterized by relatively good health, activity, and independence. These women are seeking a new flow of knowledge and a sense of being able to grow older with a purpose, in the company of peers, knowing that they are contributing and sharing within their wider community. Western society needs to provide cultural directions for older women beyond the stereotyped roles of submissive caregivers or frail recipients of care (Hewett 1993).

Clinicians play a primary role in maintaining the health and well-being of women in their later years (see Gise, Mogul, and Shapiro, Chapters 3, 6, and 7, respectively, in this volume). Many clinicians lack knowledge about women's health in general, particularly as women age (Butler 1980; Gilbert 1993; Russell 1989). The object of this chapter is to provide medical practitioners and allied health professionals with an understanding of the central issues for women as they age. We consider a broad range of issues that affect the quality of life for women as they age, including their relationships with professional practitioners, the effect of physical and psychosocial changes (see also Baram, Chapter 2, and Gise, Chapter 3, in this volume), the effect of negative attitudes and stereotyping on older women, and women's adaptive coping styles. Although the patient-clinician relationship is of importance, it does not exist in a vacuum (Sidell 1992). As such, it is important to recognize that the health and well-being of postmenopausal women continue to be of a complex and dynamic nature, and, although some degree of ill health may be experienced, it does not necessarily lead to a loss of independence or quality of life.

Diversity Versus Homogeneity

Each person is born a unique individual. As people age, they become even more individual as their experiences and personal history enhance uniqueness. The aged population encompasses a heterogeneous group with many different personal characteristics, living arrangements, and family connections (Day 1985). Aging is not a homogeneous experience that affects different individuals within the same society in the same way.

The health of women at and beyond menopause is greatly influenced by their health status in childhood, in adolescence, and through the reproductive years. Past access to health care and other services, occupations, and family history also affect the health status of older women (Kaufert 1994). Although researchers have studied older women in terms of health, income, and stereotypes, as caregivers, and in relation to family, little attention has been paid to the variations among older women (Gee and Kimball 1987; Minichiello et al. 1992). Cultural, economic, and social factors must be considered to understand the experience of aging (Sokolovsky 1993). (These factors are discussed further in Gise, Chapter 3, and Weber, Chapter 4, in this volume.)

In general, issues such as cross-cultural factors, ethnicity, and aboriginality have been neglected in relation to their effect on women and their experiences of aging (Rowland 1991). Older women whose native language is different from that of the country in which they live may have different needs than those of native speakers. It is of particular relevance that health practitioners deliver services in a way that is sensitive to cultural and language differences (American Association of Retired Persons 1991; Hanen and Williams 1989). (See Chapter 4 for further details.)

When compared with the interest shown in the experiences of and developmental patterns in children and young people, little attention has been paid to the "subtle distinctions" between age categories for people older than 60 years (Day 1985). Clinicians and allied health practitioners need to bear in mind that women's experiences vary across and within age cohorts. Clinicians should be aware that the experiences of a 65-year-old woman will be very different from those of an 85-year-old woman. They not only are from different generations but also have different experiences of, and perspectives on, aging (Gee and Kimball 1987).

Physical diversity is also present at birth but is augmented throughout the life span. Motor performance variability, for example, particularly in the aging woman, grows with each increasing decade. The variability in motor performance ranges from the frail older woman living in a care facility, who experiences severe difficulty walking, bathing, and dressing, to an 80-year-old woman living independently, who occasionally runs a 26.2-mile marathon in a masters' track meet (Spirduso and MacRae 1990).

Whether the trends that confront older women now will continue as future generations age is unclear. The older women of the future may have very different experiences and problems from those encountered by their mothers and grandmothers today. What is clear is that older women want to contribute something positive to their community, to continue to do so regardless of their age, and to be given the opportunity to develop new skills (Shanahan 1994).

Negative Stereotypes Versus Positive Images

The years for women after age 65 traditionally have been portrayed as a stage of failing health, mental incompetence, and physical deterioration. The dominant perception is that most older women will end their lives bedridden or dying alone in nursing homes (Arber and Ginn 1991; Marshall and Tindale 1978–1979). The reality, however, is somewhat different: most women remain in their own homes and live relatively independent and active lives. Clinicians must be aware of the potential that negative stereotyping and ageist attitudes have on older women. Ageism, encapsulated in statements such as "What do you expect at your age," has the potential to reduce older women's ability to maintain control over their lives, including their health and well-being (Bonita 1993). For many women, the future holds fears, and it may be difficult to stay positive in the face of the unknown. This feeling was expressed by one 72-year-old woman:

> As the years go on, if there is one paramount overriding fear it is that of being unable to be in control of one's life or one's bodily functions, a fear of being an enormous and rather revolving burden on one's children. And that I most certainly do not want to see reflected in this mirror into which I now stare. (Kamler and Feldman 1995, p. 12)

The role of the media is important in terms of constructing social views about elderly people (Anike 1991a; Gibb 1990). This role should not be underestimated because it often parodies societal stereotypes, reinforcing perceptions and misconceptions (Markson 1994). Older women are often portrayed as a "medical problem," and older women's longevity is portrayed as an indication of failure, not success (Edgar 1991; McDaniel 1986; Millar 1994). For men, the physical aspects of aging may be taken as a positive occurrence because they convey distinction, character, and status or, alternatively, maturity, experience, and power. For women in Western countries, these physical changes are not valued and, in fact, may be viewed as undesirable.

Demographic data that show increasing numbers of older women in the population are used by the media to portray older women in a negative light. An assumption made is that the aging population will put intolerable financial burden on society with substantial increases in the cost of aged care services. Older people are seen as "a drain on health resources" (Editorial 1994). However, analysis of Australian demographic data revealed that only a small proportion of women older than 65 years require institutionalization or nursing home support, and this is usually of an acute intervention rather than at a chronic level. For most older women—between 86% and 90%—assistance and support are obtained at an informal or a community-based support service level (Anike 1991b).

Very few positive images of older women are seen in film, television, and the media, and a blatant double standard exists with regard to the age and body type of women (Millar 1994). A persistent view is that women's importance lies in youthfulness and the ability to procreate. Markson (1994) wrote that dominant images of youthful and beautiful women in film reflect and reinforce the notion that older women have outlived their usefulness (Friedan 1993; Gee and Kimball 1987). This was described by one older woman participating in the pilot research project, "Women and Writing—Stories of Women and Ageing." She called her story "Past the Use-By Date":

If there's one thing that irritates me a lot it's the "use-by date." I do know that "fresh is best" and it is helpful to assess the life of the product before using it, but nothing annoys me more than when my children come home, take over the kitchen without so much as a "by your leave" study the "use-by date" in every item they pick up before devouring it or consigning it to the bin accompanied by rude remarks about aged products. We never had all this nonsense before "use-by dates" were invented and they were none the worse for it. They don't want to know anything about the pleasure of ageing wine, or brandy-ripened fruit cakes, putting down preserves or storing rich plum puddings. Some of the most delicious tastes in life frequently come after the "use-by date." (B. Kamler, S. Feldman: "Women and Writing—Stories of Women Ageing," unpublished research, August 1994)

This story illustrates that there is a crucial difference between society's image of older women and how older women experience themselves as they age. In the main, older women cope well with the aging process despite the associated physical, psychological, and emotional changes (Friedan 1993; Gee and Kimball 1987; Thompson et al. 1990; Wainrib 1992). Older women are pooling their experiences and creativity to challenge negative images that affect the quality of their lives. They are increasingly becoming consumer advocates about older people's rights rather than allowing others to advocate on their behalf (Hewett 1993).

Individuals, Families, and Society

Aging occurs within a social context ranging from the microscale of the family to the macroscale of the whole society. Baltes and Reichert (1992) claimed that successful aging is the product of biological factors, behavioral competence, and environmental quality. The biological factors are inevitable, but the other two factors may be controlled to a large extent. The behavioral competence of the individual in coping with old age is personal. At the same time, coping with old age is a particularly good measure of the quality of societal conditions in which older people age. Society needs to support and stimulate older people while providing an environment where demands and stress on older people are reduced. The years after the menopause may be characterized by disabilities, chronic ill health, poverty, loneliness, and alienation. Clinicians and health professionals must consider the implications of women's differing experiences of aging on family life, organization of work and retirement, and planning of housing and institutions (Neyland 1990).

An important element in an older woman's adaptation to aging is her relationship to family, neighbors, and wider social groups (Day 1985). Family life is an important aspect of individual well-being for women. Few women grow old in isolation, although for many, it may be a time when they live alone, most often as the result of having outlived a spouse or siblings and children who moved away. Despite the difficulty of facing the loss of a partner and the prospect of at least 7 years as a widow, a growing number of older women have emerged as an articulate and assertive group who are no longer willing to accept a passive, declining role in society.

> I was 57 at the time of his death. First came the grief, all consuming. The empty space in bed. I would put out my hand. Instead of the warm embrace it always brought on, there was cold emptiness. Then came the anger. I was angry—angry at him. Why did he leave me? (B. Kamler, S. Feldman: "Women and Writing—Stories of Women Ageing," unpublished research, August 1994)

Although some older women face diminished family responsibilities, others are the prime caregivers for aging spouses, parents, or other family members, including young children (Allen and Pifer 1993; Dalley 1993). The shift in roles is reflected in the following excerpt:

> My mother was the centre of the family, the pivot upon which everything turned, the one everyone turned to with problems to solve, worries to unload. When I visited her I could be that little girl again, just for a while. When she told me that I looked tired, I needed a rest—she would make me a nice cup of tea.
>
> In her mid-seventies, over twenty years ago, she showed the first signs of forgetfulness. She misplaced keys and bankbooks, told the same stories over and over and forgot appointments. I was not too worried, it seemed to be typical behaviour, to be expected in the elderly.
>
> It was not until several years later that I realised that my mother's behaviour was typical of sufferers of Alzheimer's disease. In a sense it was a relief; when a disease has a name and recognised symptoms, it is somehow easier to bear the fact that my clever, dependable mother has become a confused, irrational stranger. I found our roles reversed. I was now the mother and she the dependent child.
>
> For a long time she refused to leave her home, to give up what she regarded as her independence. So began the period familiar

to many children of elderly parents—travelling between her home and mine, to bring food, to make sure that she was eating, to feed the cat.

Now I am no longer young myself. I look at my mother and the other patients in the nursing home, and I can't help thinking—when will it be my turn? (B. Kamler, S. Feldman: "Women and Writing—Stories of Women Ageing," unpublished research, August 1994)

Physical Health and Well-Being

Everyone would agree that good physical health is the single most important contributor to quality of life for elderly women (Gee and Kimball 1987). The majority of older women maintain good health, although the incidence of ill health increases in the last few years of life (Bonita 1993; Rowland 1991). Although experiences with acute illnesses are less common among older persons than among younger persons, these illnesses may be more debilitating in older persons (Verbrugge 1985). Age-related and/or disease-related loss of sensory and neuromuscular capacities may be associated with a number of negative outcomes, including fractures caused by falling, dependence on others, social isolation, hypokinetic disease, and depression (see also Mogul, Shapiro, Charney and Stewart, Stotland, and Robinson and Stirtzinger in Chapters 6–10 in this volume). In contrast, the maintenance of certain physical abilities is associated with independent daily living and other markers of functional health (Greene et al. 1993). An overriding concern of elderly women is to maintain independence for as long as possible and to avoid the loss of autonomy and self-respect, which is often associated with dependence on others (Arber and Ginn 1991). Clinicians must be aware that older women judge their quality of life in terms of their ability to carry out everyday activities independently and effectively. Although good health is a key determinant of being independent and autonomous (Arber and Ginn 1991), it is incorrect to assume that some degree of ill health will necessarily result in loss of independence or quality of life.

In the past, the use of chronological definitions of age, particularly in the disciplines of geriatric medicine and gerontology, assumed that chronological age is the fundamental determinant of health and well-being, and the importance of the interaction of economic, social, cultural, and political variables was ignored. Chronological categories of aging have tended to be associated with loss of health, frailty, and overall negative images of aging and are a poor guide to functional abilities, because a wide range of disability and dependency exists within all age groups. Such categorism also has the potential to reduce the capacity of professional practitioners and social planners to respond to women as individuals, yet chronological definitions of age are evident in perceptions about the health needs of older women. These perceptions are often held by both the elderly themselves and health care providers (Gelein 1982). For example, sexual activity is often presumed to decline with age (see Lamont, Chapter 5, in this volume). Jerrome (1994) suggested that sexual expression remains important with regard to self-esteem, self-acceptance, and general well-being, particularly later in life. As one 73-year-old woman wrote, the experience of romantic sexual love came in her late 60s and after the death of her husband:

> We had the most wonderful sex. In fact I do not think that I knew what sex was all about until I met him. Quite often when I was driving away after seeing him I had to remind myself to keep my mind on the road, such was my exhilaration and joy at being with him. The amazing thing is that I have not grieved for him since his death. I am not more miserable because I cannot talk to him or see him any more. Writing about him leaves me feeling just as alive as I felt when he was here. I hope it will always be so. (B. Kamler, S. Feldman: "Women and Writing—Stories of Women Ageing," unpublished research, August 1994)

Mortality Versus Morbidity

The demographic reality is that there is a disproportionate and growing number of postmenopausal and aging women in communities around the world. The average life expectancy at birth is greater than 80 years for women and some 7 years less than that for men. However, despite their lower mortality rates, older women have greater morbidity (Barer 1994; Haug and Folmar 1986; Older

Women's League 1988; Task Force on Older Women's Health 1993). In general, older women have many of the same health problems as older men. These problems include heart disease, cancer, stroke, chronic obstructive pulmonary disease, pneumonia, and influenza (U.S. Department of Health and Human Services 1991). Older men tend to have more problems related to life-threatening conditions, such as heart disease and cancer, whereas older women report more chronic, non-life-threatening impairments (Gatz et al. 1990). Major chronic conditions in women are arthritis, high blood pressure, heart conditions, musculoskeletal problems, circulatory problems, and sensory problems (Verbrugge 1985). Clinicians are aware that many older women tend to have multiple chronic conditions, which can increase the severity of a major health condition, impose limitations on treatment strategies (Verbrugge 1985), and profoundly affect their quality of life as they age. Older women mostly live with chronic conditions rather than die from them (Verbrugge and Jette 1994). Despite this, many older women continue to play an integral role in their community and family activities.

"Use It or Lose It" Concept

Decreases in physical abilities resulting from physical inactivity, or hypokinetic disease, should be distinguished from those resulting from the aging process itself (Cunningham et al. 1993; O'Brien and Vertinsky 1991; Rikli and Edwards 1991). For years, performance declines in motor functions, such as reaction time, balance, flexibility, and grip strength, were thought to be a normal and necessary consequence of aging. Several studies, however, indicated that these declines relate more to lifelong physical activity level than to age (Rikli and Edwards 1991). With accumulated years of insufficient physical activity, people in their 30s, 40s, and 50s begin to notice a lack of physical endurance, decreased strength, increased body fat, and sagging muscles. As a result, they incorporate the feeling of "being old" into their self-concepts and participate even less in physical activity for fear of a heart attack or exercise-related injury. The decrease in physical activity produces even greater changes in body composition and more noticeable deficits in physical ability; the cycle continues as the individual exercises even less

(Berger and Hecht 1989). In the following excerpt, an active and very independent 80-year-old woman described a very severe fall that left her bruised and battered but, fortunately, without broken bones:

> At the age of 80 years is there anything more hurtful to pride than being catapulted into the air and landing on your face? Gravity! It is an ugly word. A week later the technicolour painting is still continuing, red, purple, blue black and now a dash of grey and yellow. The only thing I can do is to colour-coordinate my face— what fun. I will start a new fashion. (B. Kamler, S. Feldman: "Women and Writing—Stories of Women Ageing," unpublished research, August 1994)

In the past, most exercise studies on adults included only men, but in the last few years research about the physiological advantages of exercise for women has been undertaken (Foster et al. 1989; Hamdorf et al. 1992; Rikli and Edwards 1991). Those studies generally indicated that physical activity not only preserves cardiovascular fitness and motor functioning but also alters the adverse changes of aging. Studies also indicated that psychological improvements occur as a result of exercise in older women. These include reduction in depression (Bennett et al. 1982) and improvement in well-being (Netz et al. 1988), self-concept (Brown and Harrison 1986), and cognitive processing (Rikli and Edwards 1991).

Despite the role of physical activity in promoting health, older women have the lowest rates of physical activity of any community group (Lee 1993; O'Brien and Vertinsky 1991). Health practitioners and general society (through media and educational programs) need to develop strategies for promoting physical activity programs among older women.

Mental Health

Elderly women face mental health problems in several contexts. Depression, anxiety, self-esteem, and mood states are all emotional factors that have been extensively researched in relation to age and gender (National Health and Medical Research Council 1991) (This topic is further addressed in Chapters 3 and 8.) However, a danger is that practitioners may assume that mental disorders are related to aging, which affects diagnosis and quality of care (Butler 1980; Russell 1989). These problems may include mental health conditions that have been present over the course of a woman's life and are exacerbated by aging or by the increasing threat of the onset of dementia and Alzheimer's disease.

Depression is the single most pressing problem affecting older women's health (Dennerstein et al. 1993). Social isolation and loneliness, coupled with the devaluing of older women, are acknowledged major contributing factors to depression (Powell 1991). Researchers report that as women get older, many may face the fear of erosion of independence. This fear may be coupled with physical and mental difficulties and a reluctance to ask for help from family, public agencies, or medical practitioners (Powell 1991). The increase in physical disability for an older woman may cause anxiety and depression, which may require that drugs be administered, which in turn may lead to disability and anxiety, thus continuing the vicious circle (Bleiker et al. 1993; Gatz et al. 1990). Cattell and Wilkinson (1992) claimed that although depression is strongly associated with ill physical health, the association is nonspecific and heterogeneous with respect to physical conditions and depends largely on the affected individual's perceptions of health and personal circumstances. Newmann et al. (1990) found a rather complex pattern of symptom reporting in their sample of older women, with some symptom patterns suggesting the presence of a clinical syndrome and others suggesting milder forms of distress that may have been normal reactions to the stresses and strains of daily life. In addition to ill health and social life strains, some biological factors, particularly changes in the central nervous system, were mentioned in relation to depression. Cattell and Wilkinson (1992) also related that depression is a normal response to stressful life events such as loss of a partner, financial loss, enforced change of residence, and chronic social difficulties.

Older women living alone are more likely than women who live with husbands or partners to be poor, and anxiety about economic factors is a major concern for many single older women (Arber and Ginn 1991; Dennerstein et al. 1993; Markson 1994).

Older women who outlive spouses and friends may also experience some degree of loss and grief (Riggs and Mott 1993). However, most widows take on a new way of life without their partners, learning and accepting this change in their life pattern. They move forward into different social networks. It is important to recognize the role that social networks for older people play in preventing loneliness and isolation. Emotional well-being is, in part, a function of social interaction and the strength of social bonds (Riggs and Mott 1993). Other factors that affect older women may include barriers that prevent them from taking part in community activities because of geographical location, cultural background, or socioeconomic status (Mott and Riggs 1993). However, Barer (1994), in her analysis of gender variations in life trajectories, found some advantages for women. Many of them had experienced widowhood at a younger age, so they had time to adjust to their loss and form substitute relationships with other widows. Although many very old women have gone from strength to frailty and from self-sufficiency to some degree of dependency, their emotional and physical problems are in part counteracted by their increased social supports from children and friends.

Cattell and Wilkinson (1992) suggested that researchers should be careful not to argue that rates of depression should be higher in older women based on ageist perceptions that older women should be more depressed because of the various stressors and changes in their later years. The ageist assumption is that deterioration of physical health, increase in dependence on others, and loss of partners or neighbors through death lead inevitably to unhappiness and despair. This perspective, however, is not shared by the vast majority of older women. Usually, older women cope well with the aging process and remain active members of their community (Butler 1980; Friedan 1993; Thompson et al. 1990; Wainrib 1992).

Initiative Versus Adjustment: Developmental Theories of Advanced Age

It could be argued that in order to understand the lives of postmenopausal women it is necessary to adopt a life-course perspective. Until recently little attention was paid by developmental psychologists to the phases beyond childhood and adolescence, particularly to women in advanced age. However, contemporary research has allowed for a better understanding of the changes that take place across the life cycle (Wainrib 1992). Erikson et al. (1986) and Gutmann (1987) both sensed that late-life development has been "easily obscured by visible tangible changes in the ageing body which seems to register decay rather than growth." Yet other writers acknowledge that aging brings more realistic expectations about life and a greater knowledge of self and the world (Heaven 1992). Another woman involved in the pilot research, "Women and Writing—Stories of Women Ageing," was known for her beauty in her youth and now examines her body carefully:

> The changes must have been gradual but I did not notice. I was too busy living to see or worry about a few wrinkles and greying hair. It was not important enough. When I did notice that things had changed, I thought "I am just having a bad day, I am just tired." Then I started to examine myself and I did notice changes. (Kamler and Feldman 1995, p. 13)

Theories of life-course development have emphasized that an individual's life experiences greatly influence his or her attitude toward and experience of aging (Erikson et al. 1986; Heaven 1992). However, a limitation of life-stage theories is that many take very little account of social, environmental, or cultural contexts and, therefore, overlook the marked differences in both private and public arenas in which people live out their lives (Bernard and Meade 1993). Age may also be defined culturally and socially by expectations for appropriate behavior and by life events (Markson 1983). Although Gutmann's (1987) cross-cultural studies showed that women become more adventurous, expansive, and assertive in older years, traditional developmental theories described old age as a time for gradual reduction in life involvement, a time when meaningful roles no longer existed for the aged, much less for women. Friedan (1993) argued that these theorists have resisted confronting the fact that there is potential for further growth in old age and insisted that this trend must be overcome before it is possible to envisage new possibilities for ourselves or for society.

Professional Practice

The way health professionals relate to their older female patients is very important. Unconscious negative attitudes on the part of practitioners may lead to lack of recognition that social factors, such as isolation or poverty, affect older women's health. This may result in hurried consultation with older women or inadequate provision of information about support services (Bonita 1993).

The following clinical case vignette illustrates how financial information and appropriate grief counseling for Ms. J after her husband's death might have prevented her mental health problems.[1]

Case 1

Ms. J, a 67-year-old mother of four, was widowed some 2 years before her presentation. She presented with a moderately severe depression, which had begun suddenly 2 months previously. Features of her mental state at the time of depression included tearfulness, profoundly lowered mood, panic attacks, fears of impending doom, features of somatic anxiety, early and middle insomnia, decreased appetite, and decreased energy and concentration.

Ms. J's husband had had emphysema for many years, and she had nursed him at home for the 10 years before his death. In the course of therapy, she acknowledged that she had not mourned his death properly. She had put on a brave front for her children and others and attempted to get on with her life. The depression appeared to be precipitated by financial matters. She had always left the aspects of money management to her husband and had assumed "that he would take care of these matters properly" and that she would not have to worry about this after his death. In the months before her depression, she had been called to several meetings with the family accountant and realized that there were problems with their investments, and she was being asked to

---

[1] Most of the case vignettes cited in this chapter are from a pilot research project, titled "Women and Writing—Stories of Women and Ageing," undertaken in 1994 by one of us (Kamler and Feldman 1995). Professor Lorraine Dennerstein from the Key Centre for Women's Health in Society, University of Melbourne, Melbourne, Australia, provided two clinical case vignettes.

make decisions about matters she had never dealt with before in her life. The night before the onset of the depression, she remembered sitting bolt upright in bed and starting to cry convulsively. She thought "I'm on my own." Ms. J was unable to stay in the house by herself since this time and had gone from one relative to another. Eventually, she was brought to her local physician.

Ageism not only shapes popular perceptions of aging but also influences institutions and professional practitioners in their work with and relationships to older women (Bonita 1993; Butler 1980; Shanahan 1994). All practitioners may not have negative or ageist attitudes toward the aged, but they may have specific or treatment biases. The diagnosis of organic disorders may be influenced by a practitioner's assumptions about women as they age and may be a result of a lack of training and education with regard to normal life span development (Gatz and Pearson 1988; Kendig 1990). The biomedicalization of aging has occurred because of the tradition of viewing aging as a process of decay and decline. This is particularly relevant to postmenopausal women because aging has been viewed as a medical problem requiring medical intervention (Vertinsky 1991). Professionals are in fact trained to thrive on "cure" rather than to observe the person as a whole.

The following clinical case vignette highlights how the ill health of a partner can affect a woman's health:

Case 2

Ms. W, a 59-year-old woman, presented with complaints of nausea. She came to the appointment with her husband, age 63, who was managing director of a highly successful company. The nausea was significant enough to require the use of prochlorperazine (Stemetil). She did not complain of any other symptoms and, in particular, denied that she was depressed.

Over the last few months, Ms. W had been under a great deal of stress because her husband had had three heart attacks. She apparently feared that his working style (12- to 14-hour high-pressure days in the office) would result in his premature death, and she was very concerned that he had not altered his working style despite the heart attacks. It was also clear that her husband had not acknowledged the danger to his own life of the cardio-vascular events he had already experienced.

Further detailed questioning revealed that Ms. W had symp-toms consistent with a moderately severe depression. She had lost interest in her everyday activities, was cheerful at times, and had middle and late insomnia and nausea. She had both psychic and somatic anxiety.

The couple was encouraged to visit the cardiologist together and to take with them a series of questions. These questions in-cluded what effect the husband's continuation of current working style would have on his prognosis, and they requested detailed advice about what lifestyle he should follow to improve his prog-nosis. Ms. W's condition improved considerably with couples counseling, antidepressants, and her husband's acknowledgment of his illness and change in his lifestyle.

Professional practitioners may also view older women as de-pendent and childlike beings (Russell 1989). A recently retired 62-year-old professional woman expressed it this way:

When I arrived at 8:55 A.M. I was the first and the only client in the waiting room. The young pregnant receptionist behind the desk was offhanded. Sleepy and wishing she was still at home she re-cited the prescribed words twice, making no attempt to read the nonverbal signs of understanding, remembering the training in-junction, "Speak slowly, simply and remember that old women aren't educated, catch on slowly and may be deaf." I felt a rush of rage. The written information had explained what I already knew, and the receptionist had subjected me to yet another verbatim version. Couldn't the girl match the presentation to the person? Couldn't she see the comprehension, intelligence? Who did she think this person in front of her was, or didn't she care . . . it was just a job. (B. Kamler, S. Feldman: "Women and Writing—Stories of Women Ageing," unpublished research, August 1994)

Clinicians and health professionals also must distinguish be-tween the normal process of aging and dysfunction. Practitioners may assume that a range of disorders is related to aging, which affects diagnosis and quality of care (Butler 1980; Russell 1989). However, the boundary between normal age-related decline and disease is not entirely clear. Investigators recognize that as women enter the very old age group, physical condition declines, and, consequently, a backdrop of frailty contributes to making the individual vulnerable to a variety of diseases (Gatz et al. 1990). To date, much of the training of medical practitioners focuses on the physical problems of old age, thus reinforcing the wider negative cultural images of aging (Russell 1989). A more constructive approach would be to adopt the broad World Health Organization (1978) definition of health as a state of complete physical, mental, and social well-being and not merely the absence of disease or infirmity. Studies have found that improved training and education of health care practitioners will help to rectify this situation (Kendig 1990; Sidell 1992).

Summary

The biological process of aging cannot be stopped or reversed, and human beings are engaged in the aging process throughout the life cycle. Aging must be viewed as a continuation of, not a separation from, the earlier phases of life. The physical processes of aging may be universal, but the experience of aging for many postmenopausal women is colored by the attitudes of the society in which they grow old and by the myths and stereotypes about women, especially older women. Clinicians need to realize that women experience this stage of life in many complex and diverse ways and that the relationship between the social context and the health and well-being of older women is integral to our understanding. Clinicians must consider the role they play in maintaining the health and well-being of women beyond menopause.

For most women, the years beyond menopause have the potential to be experienced as "a new evolving stage of human life—not merely as a decline from youth but as an open ended development in its own terms, which in fact, may be uniquely ours to define" (Friedan 1993, p. 38). Increasingly, there is a recognition that older women themselves provide a positive role model. Their life experiences equip them to work in partnership with professionals to alleviate the many social problems that affect the health and quality of life of older women. The possibilities for partnership hinge on a continuing recognition by practitioners of the important role they play in promoting positive attitudes toward older women, improving communication with them, and providing accurate and up-to-date clinical information. The professional relationship between an older woman and her doctor is of paramount importance.

References

Allen J, Pifer A: Women on the Front Lines Meeting the Challenge of an Aging America. Washington, DC, Urban Institute, 1993

American Association of Retired Persons and International Federation on Ageing: Empowering Older Women: Cross Cultural Views. Washington, DC, Women's Initiative of the American Association of Retired Persons, 1991

Anike L: Challenging the myths: women and ageing. Paper presented at the University of Western Sydney, New South Wales, Australia, September 1991a

Anike L: Women over 60 growing old. Refractory Girl 39:7–9, 1991b

Arber S, Ginn J: The invisibility of age: gender and class in later life. Sociological Review 39(2):260–291, 1991

Baltes MM, Reichert M: Successful ageing: the product of biological factors, environmental quality, and behavioural competence, in Health Care for Older Women. Edited by George J, Ebrahim S. Oxford, UK, Oxford University Press, 1992, pp 237–256

Barer BM: Men and women aging differently. Int J Aging Hum Dev 38(1):29–40, 1994

Bennett J, Carmack MA, Gardner VJ: The effect of a program of physical exercise on depression in older adults. The Physical Educator 39:21–24, 1982

Berger BG, Hecht LM: Exercise, aging, and psychological wellbeing: the mind-body question, in Aging and Motor Behavior. Edited by Ostrow AC. New York, Benchmark Press, 1989, pp 117–157

Bernard M, Meade K (eds): Women Come of Age: Perspectives on the Lives of Older Women. London, Edward Arnold, 1993

Bleiker EM, Van Der Ploeg HM, Mook J, et al: Anxiety, anger, and depression in elderly women. Psychol Rep 72:567–574, 1993

Bonita R: Older women: a growing force, in New Zealand's Ageing Society: The Implications. Edited by Koopman-Boyden P. Wellington, New Zealand, Daphne Brasell, 1993, pp 189–212

Brown RD, Harrison JM: The effects of a strength training program on the strength and self-concept of two female age groups. Res Q Exerc Sport 57:315–320, 1986

Butler A: Ageism: a foreword. The Journal of Social Issues 36(2):8, 1980

Cattell H, Wilkinson G: Depressed mood in older women, in Health Care for Older Women. Edited by George J, Ebrahim S. Oxford, UK, Oxford University Press, 1992, pp 149–159

Cunningham DA, Paterson DH, Himann JE, et al: Determinants of independence in the elderly. Can J Appl Physiol 18:243–254, 1993

Dalley G: Caring: a legitimate interest of older women, in Women Come of Age: Perspectives on the Lives of Older Women. Edited by Bernard M, Meade K. London, Edward Arnold, 1993, pp 106–125

Day A: We Can Manage—Expectations About Care and Varieties of Family Support Among People 75 Years and Over. Melbourne, Australia, Institute of Family Studies, 1985

Dennerstein L, Astbury J, Morse C: Psychosocial and Mental Health Aspects of Women's Health. Melbourne, Australia, Key Centre for Women's Health, University of Melbourne, 1993

Edgar D: Ageing, everybody's future. Family Matters 30:14–19, 1991

Editorial: The coming crisis in the welfare state. The Age, Melbourne, Australia, May 2, 1994

Erikson E, Erikson J, Kivnick H: Vital Involvement in Old Age—The Experience of Old Age in Our Time. New York, WW Norton, 1986

Foster VL, Hume GJE, Byrnes WC, et al: Endurance training for elderly women: moderate vs low intensity. J Gerontol 44:M184–M187, 1989

Friedan B: The Fountain of Age. London, Random House, 1993

Gatz M, Pearson C: Ageism revised and the provision of psychological services. Am Psychol 43:184–188, 1988

Gatz M, Harris JR, Turk-Charles S: Older women and health, in Women's Psychological and Physical Health: A Scholarly and Social Agenda. Edited by Stanton AL, Gallant SJ. Washington, DC, American Psychological Association, 1990

Gee E, Kimball M: Women and Aging. Toronto, Canada, Butterworths, 1987

Gelein JL: Aged women and health. Symposium on Women's Health Issues 17(1):179–185, 1982

Gibb H: Representations of Old Age: Notes Towards a Critique and Revision of Ageism in Nursing Practice. Geelong, Australia, Deakin University, 1990

Gilbert LA: Women at midlife: current theoretical perspectives and research, in Faces of Women and Ageing. Edited by Davis ND, Cole E, Rothblum ED. New York, Haworth, 1993, pp 105–111

Greene LS, Williams HG, Macera CA, et al: Identifying dimensions of physical (motor) functional capacity in healthy older adults. Journal of Aging and Health 5(2):163–178, 1993

Gutmann D: Reclaimed Powers: Towards a New Psychology of Men and Women in Later Life. New York, Basic Books, 1987

Hamdorf PA, Withers RT, Penhall RK, et al: Physical training effects of the fitness and habitual activity patterns of elderly women. Arch Phys Med Rehabil 73:603–608, 1992

Hanen M, Williams A: Life crises and ageing people of non-English speaking backgrounds: two perspectives. Australian Journal on Ageing 8(4):3–6, 1989

Haug MR, Folmar SJ: Longevity, gender, and life quality. J Health Soc Behav 27:332–345, 1986

Heaven P (ed): Life Span Development. Marrickville, New South Wales, Australia, Harcourt Brace Jovanovich, 1992

Hewett N: Aged care—a consumer viewpoint. Paper presented at Health Services Forum, Aged Care, Tamworth Base Hospital and Health Service, New South Wales, Australia, March 3–4, 1993

Jerrome D: Sisters in later life. Paper presented at the Ageing and Gender Symposium, University of Surrey, England, 1994

Kamler B, Feldman S: Mirror mirror on the wall: reflections on ageing. Australian Cultural History Journal 14:1–22, 1995

Kaufert P: The social and cultural context of menopause. Paper presented at WHO Scientific Group Meeting, Geneva, Switzerland, June 1994

Kendig H: Challenges of change for aged care practice, in Aging Into the Nineties: Policy, Planning and Practice. Symposium Proceedings, Centre for Advanced Studies, Division of Health Sciences, Curtain University, Perth, Western Australia, 1990, pp 15–17

Kuhn M, Gray Panthers: New Life for the Elderly: Liberation from Ageism. Philadelphia, PA, Gray Panthers Tabernacle Church, 1974

Lee C: Factors related to the adoption of exercise among older women. J Behav Med 16:323–333, 1993

Markson EW (ed): Older Women: Issues and Prospects. Toronto, Ontario, Canada, Lexington Books, 1983

Markson EW: Issues affecting older women, in Promoting Successful Aging. Belmont Hills, CA, Sage, 1994

Marshall V, Tindale J: Notes for a radical gerontology. Int J Aging Hum Dev 9:163–175, 1978–1979

McDaniel SA: Canada's Aging Population. Toronto, Ontario, Canada, Butterworths, 1986

Millar M: The lady vanishes, in An Age-Old Problem or a New Opportunity: Women and Ageing. Proceedings of a public seminar at the University of Melbourne, Melbourne, Australia, The Key Centre for Women's Health, 1994, pp 41–49

Minichiello V, Alexander L, Jones D: Gerontology: A Multidisciplinary Approach. New York, Prentice-Hall, 1992

Mott S, Riggs A: Elderly people—their needs for and participation in social interactions (Research Monograph Series, Vol 5). Melbourne, Australia, Deakin University, 1993

National Health and Medical Research Council: Women and Mental Health. Canberra, Australian Government Publishing, 1991

Netz Y, Tennenbaum G, Sagiv M: Pattern of psychological fitness as related to pattern of physical fitness among older adults. Percept Mot Skills 67:647–655, 1988

Newmann JP, Engel RJ, Jensen J: Depressive symptom patterns among older women. Psychol Aging 5:101–118, 1990

Neyland B: Ageing and Death (Study Guide, Sociology of Health Care: B SSS337). Melbourne, Australia, Deakin University, 1990

O'Brien SJ, Vertinsky PA: Unfit survivors: exercise as a resource for aging women. Gerontologist 31:347–357, 1991

Older Women's League: The picture of health for midlife and older women in America. Women Health 14:53–74, 1988

Powell J: Mental health policy and older women. Refractory Girl 39:15–18, 1991

Riggs A, Mott S: The social interactions of older people—a comparative study of three communities (Research Monograph Series, Vol 8). Melbourne, Australia, Institute of Nursing Research, 1993

Rikli RE, Edwards DJ: Effects of a three-year exercise program on motor function and cognitive processing speed in older women. Res Q Exerc Sport 62(1):61–67, 1991

Rowland D: Ageing in Australia—Population Trends and Social Issues. Sydney, Australia, Longman Cheshire, 1991

Russell C: Gerontological education, research and professional practice. Australian Journal on Ageing 8(2):22–45, 1989

Shanahan P: An Optimistic Future: Attitudes to Ageing and Wellbeing Into the Next Century, Vol 13. Canberra, Australian Government Publishing, 1994

Sidell M: The relationship of elderly women to their doctors, in Health Care of Older Women. Edited by George L, Ebrahim S. Oxford, UK, Oxford University Press, 1992, pp 179–196

Sokolovsky J: Images of aging: a cross-cultural perspective. Generations 17(2):51–54, 1993

Sontag S: The double standard of aging. Saturday Review of the Society 55(23):29–38, 1972

Spirduso WS, MacRae PG: Motor performance and aging, in Handbook of Psychology of Aging. Edited by Birren JE, Schaie KW. San Diego, CA, Academic Press, 1990, pp 183–200

Task Force on Older Women's Health: Older women's health. J Am Geriatr Soc 41:680–683, 1993

Thompson P, Itzin C, Abendstern M: I Don't Feel Old—The Experience of Later Life. New York, Oxford University Press, 1990

U.S. Department of Health and Human Services: Healthy people 2000. (DHHS Publ No PHS 91-50212). Washington, DC, U.S. Government Printing Office, 1991

Verbrugge LM: An epidemiological profile of older women, in The Physical and Mental Health of the Aged Women. Edited by Haug MR, Ford AB, Sheafor M. New York, Springer, 1985, pp 41–46

Verbrugge L, Jette A: The disablement process. Soc Sci Med 38:1–14, 1994

Vertinsky P: Old age, gender and physical activity: the biomedicalization of aging. Journal of Sport History 18(1):64–80, 1991

Wainrib BR (ed): Gender Issues Across the Life Cycle. New York, Springer, 1992

World Health Organization: Alma Ata Declaration. Geneva, Switzerland, World Health Organization, 1978

Index

*Page numbers printed in **boldface** type refer to tables or figures.*

Coventry University